IF YOU LOOK AT THIN W~~OMEN WITH~~
PAINFUL PANGS OF ENVY, IF YOU THINK
LIFE WOULD BE PERFECT IF ONLY YOU
COULD LOSE FIVE OR TEN OR A HUNDRED
POUNDS . . .

you will know exactly what the women in this book
are talking about, and for the first time you will find
out what to do about it.

FEEDING THE HUNGRY HEART

*"An honest, painful, sometimes funny look at the
experience of being a compulsive eater. These
vignettes take us behind the fat, behind the so-called
greed, to the isolated and tortured struggle so many
women engage in daily and hourly with their food
and with their bodies . . . Reading these women's
experiences will be enormously helpful and liberating."*
— Susie Orbach, author
Fat Is a Feminist Issue

GENEEN ROTH, who has been both overweight and
anorexic herself, is also the author of *Why Weight?:
A Guide to Ending Compulsive Eating* and *Breaking
Free From Compulsive Eating*. She has been invited
all over the United States to conduct her Breaking
Free® workshops for compulsive eaters.

FEEDING THE HUNGRY HEART

The Experience
of Compulsive Eating

by
Geneen Roth

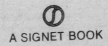

A SIGNET BOOK

SIGNET
Published by the Penguin Group
Penguin Books USA Inc., 375 Hudson Street,
New York, New York 10014, U.S.A.
Penguin Books Ltd, 27 Wrights Lane,
London W8 5TZ, England
Penguin Books Australia Ltd, Ringwood,
Victoria, Australia
Penguin Books Canada Ltd, 2801 John Street,
Markham, Ontario, Canada L3R 1B4
Penguin Books (N.Z.) Ltd, 182-190 Wairau Road,
Auckland 10, New Zealand

Penguin Books Ltd, Registered Offices:
Harmondsworth, Middlesex, England

This is an authorized reprint of a hardcover edition published by
The Bobbs-Merrill Co., Inc.

First Signet Printing, November, 1983
18   17   16   15   14   13   12   11

 REGISTERED TRADEMARK—MARCA REGISTRADA

Printed in the United States of America

To Alexandra,
for teaching me that the only way out is through

and

To Lew,
for believing in me from the beginning.

Acknowledgments

This book began the evening of my first workshop, when I had to make my appearance in curlers; the friend giving me a permanent said it was too soon to remove them. I want now to thank the ten women who came that night for not having run away—as well as every other woman since then who has come to Breaking Free and had the courage to reveal herself.

My thanks, also, to the many women who sent me their manuscripts without knowing how or when they would be used. I appreciate their patience with my delays and my general ignorance about putting this book, which is truly a collective effort, together.

Susie Orbach, in *Fat Is A Feminist Issue*, turned my vision toward a different perspective of compulsive eating. Without her book, I might still be knee-deep in a vat of ice cream and feeling guilty about every spoonful.

The individuals I want to thank for providing me with encouragement, love and chocolate along the way are: Babs Bohn, Tom Manheim and Hilary Farberow. I am especially grateful to Lucy Diggs for her help with the beginning of the book and to Tom Waggoner for his help with the final stages.

Peg Parkinson, my editor at Bobbs-Merrill, inspired me, encouraged me and pushed me to stretch myself, none of which sufficiently describes the impact she has had on my life.

Finally, my thanks to my parents; without their brimming refrigerator, this book would never have happened.

Contents

Introduction

When I was in college in Louisiana, I went on a diet a friend told me about: nothing but fried chicken for breakfast, lunch and dinner. It seemed like an unusual way to lose weight, but it sounded reasonable as well as delicious, because I had heard of the "mono-food" theory as a way of reducing. According to this approach, if you ate only one food, no matter what it was—ice cream, fudge, potato chips, bananas—you'd lose weight.

My boyfriend Lee, who was not fat but loved me very much, accompanied me on my daily search for restaurants in New Orleans that served fried chicken for breakfast. Lunch and dinner were easier. When I was five days into the diet, three pounds heavier and nauseated by the sight of anything that could have come from a chicken, the same friend who had told me about the diet came back with some unhappy news: she had gotten the story wrong. On the diet she had read about, fried chicken was the only thing you *couldn't* eat. "So sorry," she said. "I hope I didn't add to your problem."

Recently I figured out that I've gained and lost more than ten pounds thirty-five times in my life, that I've been on approximately forty-five diets, and that I've lost a total of more than five hundred pounds in seventeen years.

I am not unusual.

Every week, from ten to twenty-five women call me with similar stories. Each session of the workshops I lead, "Breaking Free from Compulsive Eating," is filled to capacity with people who have tried every procedure ever advanced for losing weight and are still uncomfortable with their bodies. Food is the pivot around which their lives revolve. Some of them don't leave the house because they are so ashamed of the way they look; some won't let anyone see them naked—they dress in the dark or behind closed doors even with a spouse; some consistently binge and throw up. All of them describe themselves as fat, no matter what their body weight. All of them dislike their bodies.

They are not unusual.

It is not news that overweight is a national obsession. According to *Goldberg's Diet Catalog*, at any given moment two hundred million people in the United States are on a diet. An estimated fifty percent of American women are overweight; and of those who manage to lose weight, between ninety and ninety-eight percent gain it back. Statistics are not available for those who are not fat but think they are, although their number is substantial.

Being and/or feeling fat is usually different for men than for women. A man can eat compulsively, be overweight, dislike his body and still be thought of—and think of himself—as attractive. A man who is twenty or thirty pounds overweight is not an outcast. He simply has a "beer belly" or a "paunch." He is not generally considered disgusting or repulsive; he does not usually have a hard time finding clothes that fit him.

On the other hand, a woman's appearance is crucial to her evaluation as a human being; a woman feels she *is* what she looks like. She may be brilliant, perceptive and competent, but if she is fat, she has to struggle to prove her worth. People stare at her; she is unable to find clothes; she is refused jobs and denied men. For a woman, overweight is synonymous with ugliness, failure and self-degradation.

I remember talking with my father one summer when I had gained ten pounds as a child; I remember crying, wanting to pull my hair out because it was so painful to live in my body. My father took me into his arms and told me that the solution was simple: all I needed to do was go on a diet. I would have to make up my mind that I didn't want to be fat; then I'd cut out sweets and starches, and that would be that; my problem would vanish. I didn't have the words then to explain my complex emotions, to tell him that it wasn't that simple.

When, a few years later, he had gained twenty pounds, I was amazed at his emotional detachment. He said he didn't like the fat and that he thought he needed to lose weight, but it was obvious that his belief in his worth as a human being was not affected. He still thought he was dashing and sexy, intelligent and capable.

Most of the men I meet and talk with about compulsive eating feel the same way; they are able to separate their *fat* from *themselves*. Women, on the contrary, view their fat as an outward sign that something is wrong with their basic nature.

I do not mean to deny that, for many men, being fat can be painful and self-depreciating. Our culture does, however, treat fat men and fat women quite differently.

Whereas I have met many men who like their bodies, men who don't even think about their bodies, I have *never* met a woman who liked her body without reservation.

Until a few years ago, it had never occurred to me that I could actually like my body *and* eat without guilt. I passed my adolescent and young adult years wishing that someone would invent an operation that could cut away half my stomach, thighs, buttocks and arms while somehow leaving my organs intact. Fascinated by thin women, I wanted to be one so badly that I would have given anything I had for a different, leggier body. I hid myself in A-line dresses and smocky maternity clothes, hoping that no one would see the outline of my hips.

In my late twenties, I gained forty-five pounds and gave up my profession. This left me with a fat body and a lot of time. I decided then that if I did nothing else for the rest of my life, I would deal with and resolve my obsession with food. Since my focus on food and the ugliness of my body pervaded my relationships, my writing, my motivation to work (even when I once weighed only ninety-two pounds), I reasoned that if I dealt with the food factor, other areas of my life would also be affected in a positive way. I was tired of waiting to be thin so that I could have a rich and meaningful life.

I began by accepting myself. I began by looking in the mirror and saying, "There might be more weight there than you want, but that's you." Then, even though I didn't believe it at the time, I added, "You're beautiful." I also began keeping daily track of my feelings as they related to my eating patterns, probing deeply into associations with food.

Most striking to me was the connection between what I did to myself physically and its emotional correlation. I began to see that I couldn't hate my body *and* appreciate myself, that one was a reflection of the other. I saw that eating was *not* the problem. And that by treating it as if it were—by dieting, depriving myself, hating my body—I was treating symptoms without working on their cause. I saw that I needed to work from the "inside out," from my feelings, my dreams, my angers, rather than from the "outside in," which began with my body. Being fat, it seemed, was fulfilling certain needs, and unless I dealt with those needs, I could lose weight many times and gain it back just as often in order to continue meeting those needs. I learned that I couldn't take away compulsive eating unless I replaced it with understanding and acceptance.

After a few years, my body reached a weight that it and I are now comfortable with. Food became a source of physical nourishment and lost its appeal when I wasn't hungry. Although occasionally I feel the desire to eat compulsively—and do—I am acutely aware that what I am wanting is not food.

After working with people individually and in groups for ten years, and doing some writing without trying to be published, I set up the Breaking Free workshops and wrote this book as a way of integrating my experience with my skills.

What moves and disturbs me about compulsive eating is the emotional damage that people inflict upon themselves; the self-hatred that festers in their guts. And the fact that most people, firmly convinced that what they lack is determination, will never know any other way of living with themselves.

This book is about recognizing, dealing with and resolving compulsive eating. It is also about the agony, the frustration, and the disillusionment of feeling and being fat.

Most compulsive eaters hide their feelings as well as their food. They don't speak to anyone about the landscape of the obsessed world they live in. They eat cottage cheese in public and ice cream behind locked doors. They feel utterly alone in what they are sure is their crazy, self-destructive world.

This book is an attempt to heal that isolation and pain. Although there has been an abundance of material on overeating and overweight published in the last few years, the *experience* of the compulsive eater remains untold. What does it feel like to eat and eat and not be satisfied? To lose twenty pounds and then to gain it back? To want not to leave the house? To throw up after every meal? What is the hunger truly about? Written by women who have struggled with the problem themselves, this book speaks graphically and with integrity about feelings and events it is difficult to talk with anyone about.

Anyone who is compulsive about *anything* will find him or herself in *Feeding the Hungry Heart.* Having worked with smokers and drinkers in Breaking Free, I know that compulsions, though they manifest themselves differently according to personality, spring from a common source: the hunger of the heart—attempting to satisfy, express, and, at the same time, numb itself. The compulsion is the individual's language; it speaks in different ways of different hungers, for different people. And this is the hunger, whether it be rooted in frustrated relationships or unexpressed emotions, that needs to be recognized and dealt with before any compulsion—eating, drinking, smoking—can be permanently resolved.

It is my hope that this book will speak to and provide nourishment for hungry hearts, in whatever language is theirs.

Geneen Roth
Santa Cruz, California
1982

Is There Life After Chocolate?

Chocolate is no ordinary food. It is not something you can take or leave, something you like only moderately. You don't *like* chocolate. You don't even *love* chocolate. Chocolate is something you have an *affair* with.

My friend Joanna told me of sitting at her kitchen table one afternoon letting some chocolate ice cream slip soothingly down her throat when there was an unexpected knock at the door.

"Who is it?" she asked in a thin voice.

"The plumber, ma'am. Your husband called this morning. Seems like you have a problem with your sink."

"My God," she thought, "he can't see me eating this. Hide it. I have to hide it."

After discovering the perfect hiding place, she smoothed her hair and opened the door for the unsuspecting repairman. Though the ice cream had been very hard (Joanna liked it that way; she liked letting the soft curls of chocolate melt around the edges. She liked collecting them ever so delicately with a twirl of her spoon and then opening her mouth to let the taste explode, sending shivers down her spine), during the course of the afternoon it did what any ice cream will do—it melted. Melted and dripped and leaked onto her white-tiled kitchen floor. The plumber, as fate would have it, noticed the lake before Joanna did.

"Hey, lady," he said, "you got chocolate dripping outta your oven. You making baked alaska or something?"

"It was an innocent question," Joanna told me, "but I felt as if my husband had just walked in and found me in bed with our next-door neighbor. If it had been vanilla it might have been different—but *chocolate!* There was something so sinful about it."

Chocolate is no ordinary food. It's different from potato chips or peanuts or cookies or other morsels you covet, sneak and protect.

Chocolate makes you do things you wouldn't do under ordinary circumstances. It makes you lusty, makes you bad.

When I was decorating my house, my friend Lennie suggested that I do the bathroom walls in a hearts-and-flowers motif. "And since it's Valentine's Day," she said, "you can go to the local drugstores and have your pick of hearts." Fifty dollars and many ruffled candy boxes later, we decided on the three that would look best pasted on my bathroom wall. As we emptied the boxes into a plastic bag, we tasted each piece, deciding which were best. Sitting on the bathroom floor, we ate the round ones, the square ones, the gold-foiled ones. We ate until we could eat no more; and then, making a valiant effort at renunciation, we threw all the other pieces into the garbage, where they landed on a heap of moldy cottage cheese.

In the morning, seized again by chocolate passion, I dived into the garbage. (Lennie had declined to join me.) Retrieving the chocolate, I washed off the mold, and although the taste was a bit fermented, I again achieved chocolate saturation and went through the ritual of discarding once more.

By noon I was nauseated. When John the carpenter appeared to drop off a bill, I asked if he would like some chocolate. Yes, he said, eyes glistening, he'd love some. John knew about my reputation as Princess Truffle of Santa Cruz and was, I am sure, expecting the very best. After a short delay during which I excused myself and scurried into the kitchen, I handed him perhaps not the finest but the cleanest chocolate in town. He accepted the gift with thanks and left, treasure in hand. Lennie, in the meantime, had retreated to the bedroom, where I found her gasping in muffled mirth. "You're *bad*," she said, "very, very bad."

Some people measure their lives by styles of clothes or erstwhile lovers. I mark mine by chocolate history.

The first milestone came in fifth grade, when my teacher asked the class where we would like to go for our field trip. Of thirty-two students, fifteen chose the United Nations, sixteen chose the Statue of Liberty, and one chose Hershey, Pennsylvania.

"But why do you want to go *there?*" the teacher asked me, a touch of irritation in her voice.

"Because," I said, "I heard that the lampposts are shaped like candy bars and the whole town smells like chocolate. Not only that, but if you visit the factory, they give you free samples of chocolate bars—the ones with almonds."

Although I thought it was rather gutsy of Me—ol' Moon Face, as I was known—to stand in front of thirty-one hardware mouths extolling the virtues of chocolate, the teacher was not impressed. We went to the Statue of Liberty and I got seasick on the Staten Island ferry.

I was mad about chocolate, driven by it, passionate in the presence of a Milky Way. I still am.

It's my mother's fault. She told me that I was allergic to it. She lied.

The fact was that the backs of my legs used to break out in a terribly itchy and ugly rash. My mother blamed it on chocolate. I think it was from trying on clothes in the Chubby section of Macy's.

When my mother was young, she inhaled whole loaves of buttered bread. Consequently, *her* mother took her to the Chubby section to buy clothes. Chubby is worse than Maternity insofar as selections go: sailor suits and pink polka dots with an occasional ruffle. Lots of dark vertical stripes. Horizontal anything is never stocked. My mother, dressed as a child in pink verticals, cried a lot. When she saw her own daughter gravitating to chocolate, her visions of me in tight little horizontal suits were threatened. So she lied.

But it didn't stop me. I sneaked frozen Milky Ways into my pajamas and unwrapped the candy under the covers so no one would discover me. With my heart pounding and my head covered by quilts, blankets and bedspreads, I dived into the candy like the M&M peanut on TV.

At holiday times, boxes of chocolates flowed freely into the house. I liked the solid pieces best, but until I became an expert, it was difficult to tell which ones were filled with that disgusting cherry or pineapple and which were solid chocolate through and through. I'd make a crack at the bottom of every piece, and if it was liquid inside, I'd use the candy's juice and some spit to glue it back together. (If you think that's bad, my mother used to lick the insides of Oreo cookies, stick them together and put them back in the package. No wonder she had to shop in the Chubby section.)

When I was eighteen, I went to Europe, where I graduated from Hershey's and Nestlé's to Godiva and Perugina.

The flight from Florence to Pisa was aboard a rickety twelve-seater, a Wright Brothers model. Convinced it would never touch the earth again, I reasoned that I'd better eat the five-pound box of Perugina kisses I had bought for my mother. One by one, I methodically removed the gold and blue wrappers and popped the nougats into my mouth. "Since I'm going to die," I thought, as the taste of the kisses bathed my tongue and cheeks and filled my head with chocolate sensation, "what difference does it make that I will be fat? Isn't it just as easy to die eating chocolate than not?" I didn't walk off that plane. I rolled.

My chocolate history took a reverse turn after that. Hearing of the spirits that live in dead meat, I turned vegetarian. Not only vegetarian (the kind who doesn't eat red meat, fish or poultry) but lactotarian (the kind who doesn't eat dairy products). Not only lactotarian but raw foodatarian (the kind who doesn't eat cooked food). There wasn't, as you can imagine, much food I could eat. Protein rotted in the intestines, cooked food was deadening, and chocolate—my God, *chocolate*, who could commit such an atrocity as to eat it? It contained not only poisonous white sugar (Gloria Swanson wouldn't touch it) but milk, the deadly dairy product. Not only dairy but caffeine, the artificial stimulant. Chocolate was absolutely out of the question.

And so I choked down wheat grass and fungus health drinks, gagged on lentil and mung and azuki bean sprouts, walked around with orange-colored skin from drinking vats of carrot juice, and tolerated the ridicule of my family and friends.

One day I lay on my bed (without protein it's difficult to move) reading a book by Randolph Stone, the founder of Polarity Therapy. He wrote that "a happy person could digest a rock." I reread the sentence. "A happy person could digest a rock." My mind worked quickly: a rock was most assuredly harder to digest than chocolate. And since chocolate made me happy. . . . Within hours, I had thrown out my books on food combining, miracle fasts, and the healing properties of grapes and lemons and turned my attention once more to the food of the gods.

By this time Bloomingdale's had a Godiva department, and Haagen-Dazs had invented chocolate chocolate chip ice cream. My friend Rebecca first met a man in a New York City Haagen-Dazs store three times in one week and decided, after learning that his favorite flavor was also chocolate chocolate chip, to marry him. That was the beginning of my steadfast belief in the erotic properties of chocolate.

Drs. Donald Klein and Michael Liebowitz at the New York State Psychiatric Institute seem to agree. After extensive research on the nature of love, they say that a body in love produces a chemical called phenylethylamine. Chocolate is loaded with that very same substance.

Chocolate, I am sure, is the *concrete manifestation of love*. Not only love but lovemaking as well.

Like lovemaking, chocolate has its subtleties. One kiss comes to you shrouded in plain silver foil, another emblazoned in royal blue and gold. Some kisses fade like childhood on your mouth, while others quiver with dreams not yet conceived. Some chocolates, like some lovemakings, give you a quick heady rush and let you down before you come out the other side. Others, of both categories, allow you to build to a gradual climax, with glimmers of ecstasy along the way, until a final cry is reached and you sink into the shadow of the moon.

Streaks of chocolate penetrate your mouth, explode in fragments along your arms, move down to your fingers, through your throat and into your stomach; like tiny points of light, they awaken and revitalize each cell of your body. Chocolate electrifies your senses, shocks you into perceiving again. Like love.

And so, I ask you, is there life after chocolate?

Be truthful now.

BINGEING:
You Can Never Get
Enough of What You
Don't Really Want

"She wanted to know how I gained seven pounds
in two days. So I told her: I started the day
by going out to breakfast and then I came home and
ate breakfast. After that, I met a friend for lunch
and then took my kids out to lunch and then I
came home and fixed lunch for myself. When it came
time for dinner, I ate with my family, after the
kids were asleep, and then again in the bathtub.
At midnight, I had a snack in front of the TV.
When I woke up in the middle of the night, I
had a different snack. The next day I followed
the same schedule.

"That's how I gained seven pounds in two days.
It was easy."

—a *Breaking Free workshop participant*

I.

I was in high school, eleventh grade. It was in the late sixties. My friend Marilyn and I had a "sleep-over" date at my house; my parents and brother were going out, so no one would be home. Late that afternoon, we went to a local delicatessen and bought fried chicken breasts, shrimp salad, crab meat salad, potato pancakes, knishes, stuffed cabbage and rice pudding. Next we stopped at the local ice cream hangout and asked the man to hand-pack three of our favorite flavors. In the empty house, Marilyn and I opened all the bags, the plastic containers, the pints of ice cream, and put them on the kitchen table. We filled our plates with an assortment of food, then went into my parents' bedroom, turned off the lights and switched on the television set. At every commercial, we would hurry back to the kitchen, pile up our plates again and return to lie on the bed in the darkened room, slurping, crunching, gulping our way through one plate after another. We moaned and sighed in mutual satisfaction, our eyes gleaming. Conversation would have been a distraction; our focus was food, the speed at which we could cram it in and down. We were accomplices in crime; we were doing what was most forbidden: eating exactly what we wanted and as much of it as we pleased.

After a few hours of uninterrupted chewing and swallowing, our stomachs were so distended that no bodily position felt comfortable. We wrapped up the remnants of the food and threw them away, being careful to leave no evidence of our transgression, our flight into sensuality. My mother, I was sure, upon smelling of the skin of the chicken or discovering a smear of rice pudding, would be angry; she already thought I was too fat.

Marilyn and I slept fitfully. We awoke with a binge hangover: the peculiar but familiar sensation of empty fullness. We never talked about that night, not the morning after, not ever. (We were, I think, both glad for and ashamed of our actions. Beyond that, we had no words for what we had done or why.)

For years I used that escapade and all the binges before and after as proof to myself of my craziness around food. Other binges weren't so calculated or so much "fun" (I usually binged alone); they were desperate acts punctuated by hysteria and self-hatred.

When I was twenty-six, I decided to be a doctor. While I was taking the science courses I needed in order to apply to medical school, I spent my afternoons roaming from one health-food store to another, digging my hands into the tubs of carob-coated peanuts, yogurt malt balls, and tamari roasted nuts, and shoving as many into my mouth as I could without getting caught. After my grocery cart was filled and I was certain no one I knew was in the store, I'd go to the checkout counter and pay for my purchases and go home. Once inside the door, I'd take the phone off the hook, close the curtains, and sit in the middle of my kitchen floor, eating from each bag in turn. I'd eat until I got sick, until I cried from desperation and self-loathing. Then I would force myself to study chemistry, physics, and calculus until I'd fall asleep exhausted.

II.

The inside of a binge is deep and dark; it is a descent into a world in which every restriction you have placed on yourself is cut loose. The forbidden is obtainable. Nothing matters—not friends, not family, not lovers. Nothing matters but food. Lifting, chewing, swallowing—mechanical frenzied acts, one following the other until a physical limit, usually nausea, is reached. Then comes the sought-after numbness, the daze, the indifference to emotional pain. Like a good drug, food knocks out sensation.

A few years ago, when I was caught in the eye of my worst eating days, I wrote: "I feel so insane when I binge, as if there is no reality but the loud pounding voice inside my head screaming at me to eat. At that moment nothing else exists; yet, because I am so aware that everything else does in fact exist, the contrast and craziness of what I am doing make the insanity even sharper. I *know* I am destroying myself, but I can't stop. I am so driven at that point that no one I know would recognize me. In those moments, the darkness is so pervasive that it is as if I have descended into another realm. When I surface and see that other people are here, that there is actually sunlight and words, that the bougainvillea outside my window is budding with tiny white insides, I feel infinitely relieved—and then even more shattered for having just experienced a thirty-minute frenzy, a dive into hell."

At the core of a binge is deprivation, scarcity, a feeling that you can never get enough.

III.

Binges are purposeful acts, not demented journeys. They do not signify a lack of willpower or the inability to care for yourself. On the contrary, a binge can actually be an urgent attempt to care for yourself when you feel uncared for.

Binges speak the voice of survival. They are protective mechanisms. Binges are signals that something is terri-

bly wrong, that you are not giving yourself what you
need—either physically (with food) or emotionally (with
intimacy, work, relationships). They are your last stand
against deprivation.

You binge on foods that you don't otherwise allow
yourself to eat. Something that is being forbidden is
needed by the body or the psyche, and a binge is your
way of letting yourself know. If deprivation worked, binges
would not be necessary. Binges are valuable messages;
they are worth listening to.

Bingeing is the only way many of us know how to give
to ourselves without holding back. Binges are acts of
rebellion. They are the mark of the self that says, "I am
tired of feeling deprived, of being told I am wrong, that I
am bad. I am tired of constant restrictions. Go to hell."

As painful as they are, they serve an important function in the binger's life. Aside from being the direct line to
a self that is calling out to be valued, they provide emotional release from situations that are difficult to handle.

In January of my junior year in high school, my first
love, a boy named Sheldon, died of a rare kind of cancer.
By June I had gained twenty-five pounds, and my grief at
his death had been replaced by overwhelming misery at
the size of my body. Years later, in my health-food-store
period, bingeing allowed me to take the focus off my
abhorrence of chemistry and physics and my doubts
about having chosen to be a doctor. Bingeing is such an
emotionally frenetic activity that no other concerns can
exist in the same space. It is a hell that people who are
food-sensitive are familiar with; and, because it is known,
it is therefore not so terrifying as some of the problems
that are outside our control. Problems like divorce, illness,
death.

IV.

When I first begin working with people in my groups, they tell me that who they are and what they feel are wrong. This feeling is the foundation on which everything else is built.

If who you are is wrong, then what you want is also wrong. If what you want is wrong, you must constantly be on guard against yourself, depriving yourself, never giving yourself what you want because that's also wrong; you can't be trusted. The fear is that if you allowed yourself to *be* yourself, you would devour the whole world. And on an emotional level, if you let yourself be yourself, no one would love you.

The antidote to this feeling of essential wrongness has to do with a mixture of forgiveness, acceptance and the cultivation of self-trust; the antidote to deprivation is the cultivation of abundance, both literal and figurative.

Imagine yourself going to the grocery store with an unlimited amount of money to spend and choosing all the foods you want, all the foods you have not allowed yourself to eat. Imagine yourself filling your kitchen with the foods you love, tasting and eating them. Stay with yourself—notice the fear, the dread, the exhilaration of being surrounded by foods you crave. Notice what it feels like to give yourself what you want. By giving attention to a voice of trust and confidence that has been heretofore ignored, you can start nurturing your self-respect.*

Buy one "forbidden" food a week. Eat it when you are hungry and when you want it. Over and over, give yourself the message that you need not deprive yourself, that you can be trusted to care for yourself. You will probably

---

*My thanks to Susie Orbach in *Fat Is a Feminist Issue* for the suggestion of this fantasy.

have to do this many times in order for your voice of "essential wrongness" to hear you.

In time your bingeing will cease. It will drop away slowly, almost imperceptibly, as you start giving yourself what you need in ways other than with food. It will not happen forcefully or with pressure; the process is natural, evolving as your self-concept changes. After a while, you will realize that you haven't binged in six months, nine months, a year. When you are no longer depriving yourself, the need to binge drops away. As a snake molts its last year's skin, you step out of your bingeing because it has outlived its usefulness.

During the first session of a workshop I led, one of the women told the group that food was the drug of her choice. She said that what a binge meant to her was concentrating on one food and eating it for long stretches of time with short intervals of rest. "I have some pain," she said, "after I eat continuously for an hour, but then it subsides and I can start eating again."

I suddenly realized that I hadn't binged in two years. I remembered the days of my own bingeing, and I was struck by the feeling of giddy relief that marked the onset of each of my binges. I remembered Marilyn's face, my laughter, the vigor with which I had bitten into the chicken.

The pain of Sheldon's death had been overwhelming to me. I didn't know what to do with it or myself, how to make sense of the rage, the grief, the hollowness I felt. I remember thinking I would never laugh again. A month later, I was exhilarated by my decision to binge. I handled Sheldon's death by eating continuously for six months; the food afforded me relief.

These days I sleep or write or ask someone to hold me.

The problem with bingeing is that the relief is only temporary.

When it's all over, the pain that you binged about is still there.

I tried to make death go away. I wooed it with fried chicken and crab salad, tried to smother it with rice pudding. But six months and twenty-five pounds later, the pain was still there.

Congratulations, Barbara! A Little Something for My Toothless Friend

I admit it: I'm a liar. Not by choice, I can assure you, but for self-preservation. As a fat woman it isn't easy to be out in the world trying to eat the things I want to eat. Everywhere eyes are staring. People are judging. How can I walk into a bakery and order cookies from a skinny blonde who looks like the last time she ate was the spring of '75?

So I have happened on a few methods, tried and true, to sneak by the slender juries of the marketplace. There are ways of obtaining food so that the only people who know I am really going to eat it myself are me and Judge Detecto (my scale).

I divulge below a few secrets:

—Go to a bakery and order a large cake to be prepared with the inscription: CONGRATULATIONS, BARBARA! Actually, the name "Elizabeth" might be better, because it takes more frosting to spell it.

—Go to a different bakery. Don't even look in the

display case. Take out a piece of paper and read from it: "I need six eclairs, six creme puffs and six napoleons." Always say "need," not "want." Act very rushed and businesslike.

—Go to 31 Flavors. Ask them if they have kumquat sherbet. When they say no, look disappointed and sigh. "I guess I'll just have to get jamoca almond fudge, but little Bobby really wanted kumquat."

—Go into See's Candy. Order one chocolate-covered peanut cluster while you wait for the clerk to hand-pack two pounds of all cream centers. Keep checking to make sure she doesn't put anything with nuts in the box. Explain your anxiety: "My friend has no teeth."

—Visit another chocolatier. Order ten truffles and ask if they have any Happy Cinco de Mayo paper. When they look at you in a peculiar way, act forgiving. Say lightly: "Oh, well, Juanita would have probably just ripped it open anyway. She gets like that around chocolate, you know."

—Call a pizzeria. Ask what size pizza you should order for ten people. If they answer "extra large," order two extra larges and tell them you expect your friends will all bring dates. (This will not be questioned in our couplistic society.)

—Go into a gourmet cheese shop—you know, the kind that smells like a yeast infection? Hide behind a large gruyère and yell FIRE! When everyone runs out, fill your backpack with little things to eat. Don't forget marmalade.

—Go into Walgreen's and ask where the Rolaids are. After such a successful round of shopping, you'll need them.

—*Ronda Slater*

Sugar and Spice

Marge Smith is closing the door, the heavy wooden door, and locking all three locks. The teeth of the top lock bite down. Closed. Tight. The middle lock—a quick turn to the left. Done. The chain lock nudged gently into place across the crack in the door. She is safe and alone. She begins to empty the grocery bag. Escarole—green camouflage—she drops it onto the counter. She tosses peppers, cucumbers, tomatoes out of the bag onto the kitchen table. A pepper rolls over the edge onto the floor, lodges against the leg of a kitchen chair. In the bottom of the bag, hidden, she has two quarts of Haagen-Dazs chocolate chocolate chip ice cream, fudge, syrup, walnuts, Reddi-Wip in a can, and maraschino cherries.

Mr. Olivero from the apartment upstairs had met her on the steps, his umbrella tapping in front of him. "Good day, Miss Smith," he had said, his dark eyes narrowing as he smiled. A portly gentleman, Mr. Olivero; curled moustache, greased-down hair. He had stood to one side of the staircase as she approached. Barely room for her to pass. She had shrunk toward the wall, moving carefully around his protruding stomach.

Tap. Tap. She can still hear the umbrella against the bottom steps. Then the slamming front door. From somewhere out on the street comes the sound of a transistor radio, children calling out to each other.

She is certain Mr. Olivero didn't notice the ice cream

and syrup. The escarole leafing from the top of the bag would have hidden everything underneath.

Marge pulls the top from the ice cream container and licks the chocolate from the underside. A spoon. She chips away at the block of ice cream, one small piece at a time. Easier to run the container under hot water, carefully from side to side, until the whole quart slides into a mixing bowl. Her treat for herself. She has been good all day—and yesterday. No salad dressing at lunch. Not even one spoonful from the big boat of blue cheese dressing with floating lumps of cheese. She'd taken a hard-boiled egg instead. Seventy-five calories. Protein.

"Oh, you're so virtuous," her co-worker Madeline had said to her with a sigh as she added a roll and butter to her own tray. Slender Madeline in a short-sleeved blue dress that showed off her well-muscled arms, her narrow hips.

Immediately after lunch Marge had begun to feel a gnawing emptiness in her stomach. The night before, she'd had only a small piece of roast chicken, cabbage salad, string beans, then a glass of skim milk before bed. For breakfast—black coffee. She'd thought all afternoon about food—mocha cheesecake, cinnamon apple coffee cake, chocolate chip cookies warm from the oven. The idea of food in her mouth made her feel light-headed and weak, until there were so many mistakes in the letters she was typing for Mr. Osgood that she'd had to stay late making corrections.

Mr. Osgood had waited for her to finish. He'd stood next to her typewriter, looking down at his watch, sighing with annoyance, pacing back and forth in front of her desk. She could feel him watching her. Her fingers were shaking. She'd begun to perspire. She could hardly breathe.

"Are these all right?" she'd asked timidly as she handed

the letters up to him. The changed characters stood out darker than all the others against small, blurred patches of white. He stared at the letters, then at her, then back at the letters.

"I suppose they'll have to do, won't they?" he said and bent down to her desk to scrawl his name across the bottom. He pushed them toward her. "Make sure these go out in tonight's mail," he said. He picked up his briefcase, turned sharply on his heel and walked out, slamming the door behind him.

Marge leaned her head against the typewriter. She felt tired, sweaty. Hunger was a distinct pain now. Her mouth began tingling as she thought of the sensation of cold chocolate. She could imagine biting down into the small, hard pieces of chocolate chip.

Marge runs her spoon along the sides of the block of Haagen-Dazs chocolate chocolate chip in the mixing bowl. It's softer, melted now. She looks around for the can opener, punches two large holes in the chocolate syrup container. Half for now, half for later, she thinks, pouring the syrup over the top of the ice cream. She dips into the chocolate mound, bringing up a creamy dark spoonful. Whipped cream. She discards the top of the Reddi-Wip can, pushes hard on the rubber neck. Whipped cream forms in puffy clouds under her fingers, slides down the sides of the ice cream until nothing can be seen of the chocolate except a dark pool around the bottom of the bowl. Walnuts. She rips open her cellophane bag, puts a handful in her mouth, pours more atop the whipped cream. They sink softly into the white mounds. A cherry for the top. One for her now. The sweet taste of maraschino fills her mouth as she bites the cherry in half.

She had intended to buy only the ice cream. Three hundred calories a half cup. Fattening, but she would eat nothing else. She'd been so tired, so hungry. Mr. Osgood staring at her. She'd felt herself growing light-headed, dizzy.

In the supermarket she hadn't gone immediately to the ice cream counter. Instead she'd looked hopefully at the rows of citrus fruit, picked up a grapefruit and prodded it to see whether it was firm all around. No use. All the while she was thinking of chocolate. She put the grapefruit back and began to wheel her cart toward the frozen foods. She paused again opposite the escarole. She would be embarrassed to have only ice cream in her shopping cart. People would stare at her. Overweight, they'd say to themselves. No self-discipline. Weak. Her beige suit, the bulky jacket, the straight skirt didn't hide anything. The skirt was too tight and pulled uncomfortably across her hips. Her stomach protruded below the waistband. Marge pulled her shoulders back, her stomach in.

There was a crash from one of the aisles. Marge jumped. "No!" she heard a woman's voice. "I told you, you can't have any. You've been a bad boy." A small blond-haired child stood in a shopping cart crying. On the floor lay several boxes of Oreo cookies. His mother bent over to pick them up. The little boy watched her, tears streaming down his cheeks. "I'll teach you to behave," his mother said, fitting the cookies back into their neat row on the shelf. She gritted her teeth. "You're going to get it." She reached in and shook him roughly by the shoulders. The child set up a wail of distress.

Marge began to load up her cart with vegetables—the escarole, peppers, cucumbers, tomatoes. She took whatever was on top. May as well hurry, she thought to herself. She would hide the ice cream safely in the bottom of a grocery bag until she got home.

She pushed her cart toward frozen foods, past the

canned fruit juices, the packaged vegetables, the TV dinners. Just ahead were the rows of Haagen-Dazs. She slowed down a little to let a woman shopper make her choice among the flavors. The woman leaned far over the freezer. Such thin hips. Directly above the ice cream were toppings—pineapple, marshmallow, strawberry and chocolate.

Mouthful after mouthful. No stopping, not even to sit down. Marge stands at the kitchen counter tasting the cold, rich chocolate, the sweet whipped cream melting into it. Just this once, she tells herself. Something to make her feel better. The hungry emptiness in her stomach is disappearing, but the tingling sensation is still on her tongue. Outside she can hear children's voices, louder now, screaming.

"That's enough," she says to herself out loud. "You're not hungry any longer." She looks down at her stomach, then at her thighs. So large. She runs her hands down the sides of her hips and pushes down hard against the flesh. In front of a mirror she examines her face. Cheeks puffy and round.

"Look at you," she says to her face in the mirror. She turns around to stare at herself over her shoulder. Her skirt seems to pull more tightly across the rounded mass of her hips.

The stairs. Someone is coming up the stairs. The footsteps seem to stop outside the door. Marge looks around her. Ice cream still in the mixing bowl, the torn container on the counter. Escarole, vegetables strewn everywhere. Walnuts in the open bag. Maraschino cherries with the lid off the jar. Too much to clear away if someone is at the door. Her mouth feels cold. No one can come in here now, she thinks. The room has grown dark. No one can tell that she is home.

That time long ago. She remembers. Her parents'

house. They'd lain so still on the sofa, she and Dan. She could feel her heart pounding. His kisses, his tongue slipping between her teeth. She'd taken her blouse off; his hands were caressing her breasts. Her skirt halfway up her thighs. Suddenly the sound of a key in the lock. The door opened. They were home already, back early. She looked up. Her mother frowned. Her father's eyes were small narrow slits.

The footsteps continue upstairs. Marge can hear them stop outside an apartment on the floor above, can hear the keys in the locks. A door closes.

She starts to breathe again. The sweet taste of ice cream is still in her mouth. The sundae is exactly as she likes it now, all the flavors of chocolate and cream melting together. The nuts softer, no longer hard to bite. But she's not hungry anymore. So full. She feels so full. The spoon falls into the streaked pool of whipped cream at the bottom of the bowl. She feels sleepy. The dark room closes around her. The street noises grow dim.

Outside she can hear the tinkling sound of the Good Humor bell. She smiles. So little they give you, she thinks. One small bar of chocolate-covered ice cream on a stick.

"One is enough," her mother would say, looking down at her with disapproval. "Too many sweets and you'll be sorry."

Marge sinks into the cushions of her sofa. The hunger is gone. She can forget about Osgood and his letters and all the rest. She is safe now and alone.

—*Sylvia Gillett*

Sunday, 4:30 p.m.

What is it about overeating that makes me want to take a
bath? I don't mean the kind of overeating one does at a
six-course restaurant meal, with friends. I can get through
one of those all right, and usually top it off with a piece of
cheesecake or a cup of tea and a good deal of laughter.
No, I mean the kind of overeating one does alone, or at
least I do alone, when I'm bored, or tired, or anxious, or
lonely. The kind that starts out with one cookie and ends
up seven cookies, two sandwiches, two glasses of milk,
three frozen cupcakes, several chunks of cheese, and
four pickles later. The kind that leaves you with a stomach so stretched that the hurt is like fingernails scratching over the skin of a too-tight balloon. Right then, at that
balloon point, I always want to get into the tub.

And I usually do. I have most of my eating binges in
my own kitchen. Finished, I climb the stairs and start the
water running, testing with my hand until it is as hot as
flesh can tolerate. Submerged in the painful yet comforting heat of the water, I soak until my skin reddens and
sweat beads up on my face. When I think I cannot stand
another second, I count to sixty slowly, forcing myself to
stay a minute more. Then to bed, where I lie wet and
naked under the covers while the pounding of blood
through my veins flushes the fat feeling out of my body.

It is fifteen minutes before the pounding stops completely and longer yet before I can get up, dress, and
reenter the civilized world.

There is so much torture in that process that it becomes almost a baptism. It is a ritual for me now; I've performed it a hundred times or more. Does the bath give me a chance to try again and to start the trying clean?

—*Carolyn Janik*

For You

Having at the moment more time for shopping than you do, I stop by the bakery, hoping the woman I enjoy talking with or her bearded Jewish husband is behind the counter. There is no bread in the kitchen, and a new loaf would be a nice treat for you when you return home late and tired. Crisp with melted butter, laid on a plate passed to you—it would bring a smile, I know.

He is there, Old World man, aproned and smiling his knowing smile. There are two whole-meal loaves—wholemeal, much better for you—one regular and one shining round, dark brown. Both the same price, same weight. ("Of course; government regulations.") I choose the special one.

Carrying the tissue-wrapped loaf, I return home, put the package inside the breadbin in the kitchen down the hall, and get back to my unstructured writing work.

The bread begins to assert its existence; visions of the crisp crust enclosing nutritive, natural, good-for-your-body elements float in and out . . . from down the hall and all about. Being a sensitive, receiving person, I respond.

The serrated red-handled bread knife carefully cuts through an end piece. It's soft, chewy, crunchy. All textures combined in one bite. Bliss. All in only one small slice.

The loaf looks better after it's been cut into. You can see the form—decide how it will be sliced.

It has rye seeds in it, I think.

I didn't use any butter. You buy Irish butter. I use margarine, even diet margarine if I can find it in London stores. The knife is still out, lying close to the breadbin. I'll just slice off a small rounded piece on the other side and try it with your special butter. It will be much different from plain bread.

It is. It adds smooth to the soft chewy crunchy. So nice. So nourishing. So substantial. Not like the mushy airy roll-in-a-ball between your fingers slices of white bread. I can almost feel the vitamins, the fiber being ingested. So healthy. Now I have the energy to work.

Hot tea would be nice. I put the kettle on and wait. No sense returning down the hall, since I'd just have to turn around and come back. A watched pot never boils. Dum de dee, de dum. I could try a thin, a very thin slice without crust while I'm standing here . . . with butter.

Tea's done, and I return to my work at the table with the hot cup. Type and think. Type. Stare out the window. Rain forming puddles with bubbles on the top. Lorries rumbling by. Clouds. Dreary gray. Finished with the tea, I decide that leaving a dirty cup around your place is not a good idea. I return it to the kitchen, where the living dark loaf shines out through the closed rounded breadbin.

There's a lot of crust there. In retrospect, I don't think you like crust at all. I remember your leaving pieces of it on plates in the past. All that crust. I cut carefully from the third side. Now there are three square sides and one rounded. It certainly doesn't look aesthetically balanced.

Perhaps if I just cut off the last rounded side . . . I really think you'll be glad that no piece has a lot of crust.

There. It looks more normal. Now it won't be a suspect renegade loaf in your mind. I wonder, though, whether you will question how it came to look like this.

My writing isn't coming too easily. Maybe I am no writer of reports. This is the culmination of three terms of research, three terms of thinking. So much to get down. Others will be reading it; but more than that, I will be reading it. Let's see, the beginning. Always hard, that.

You know, I could cut off the top of the loaf. It's almost all crust. Great idea. The faithful red-handled accomplice is waiting. Slice through. No butter this time. Ahhh. Great idea. Now back to the report.

Oh, what the heck, I've eaten most of it. I bet that bottom part would be fantastic. It looks even more crusty and chewy than the rest. It would be sort of the culmination of the loaf . . . its essence. Besides, I will have to come up with some explanation of this thing, this odd loaf, for you.

The bottom, with butter, was terrific. The way I cut it left almost no soft bread on the slice. The loaf is a perfect rectangle now. Of course, it will be a little awkward to explain how this loaf came about. It looks naked there, vulnerable, with no top, bottom, sides.

Luckily for my proper pride, you aren't interested in perusing your food supplies, because there in the breadbin sits the exposed center of a loaf of black bread. I think I can toast it for you in the morning when you're not too alert anyway. There should be no noticeable evidence of overwhelming crust consumption in a groggy early-morning glance.

Yes, for breakfast I'll fix some eggs with black bread toast—sustaining black bread bought just for you.

—Janet Robyns

BODY IMAGE
Being and/or Feeling Fat

"If Jane Fonda, upon spending time with Katharine Hepburn, found herself wanting to become her (Hepburn), whaddya think it feels like in my body?"

—*a Breaking Free workshop participant*

"I have so many voices pulling at me. One voice tells me to diet, another says diets are too restricting. One voices tells me to fast and another tells me to binge. I get very hungry listening to all these voices and then I have to eat. And I have to eat a lot because it's not just me I'm feeding, it's all these other voices, too."

—*a Breaking Free workshop participant*

Dr. Colby was tall, with stiff gray hair and a head that wobbled when he walked. He thought I was too fat. He told me that a lot, but especially each June, when I had to go to him for my camp physical.

On the day before the physical, our maid, Ann, would spend the afternoon with me as I stepped in and out of steamy baths, trying to melt the pounds away. After each bath I'd weigh myself, with Ann putting her head over my shoulder to peer at the scale. "A few more pounds," I'd tell her, "and I'll be okay." So we'd draw another bath and she would sit with me as the beads of perspiration formed on my face and my fingertips grew shriveled. When I couldn't stand the heat anymore, we'd leave the bathroom and spend the next hour or so doing exercises on the pink shag carpet in my bedroom. Ann watched Jack LaLanne on television every morning, so she was well versed in the latest and most uncomfortable calisthenics for waist, hips and thighs.

She would insist that I eat half a grapefruit and a soft-boiled egg mashed with spinach for dinner. One year, she heard that if you ate grapefruit before the meal, it burned up the caloric content of the rest of the meal; the next year the theory changed, and grapefruit, in order to serve its function as a fat burner, had to be eaten at the end of the meal. Chronology aside, the meal was always the same. When I was through, she'd go home and I'd go to bed. By the next morning my nerves were stretched taut. I'd walk down the block to Dr. Colby's, thinking, "In an hour it will be over. Tonight it will be over. In an hour I'll be free." One year I threw up Sugar Smacks outside his door.

Every visit was the same. I'd have to take off all my clothes except my panties. He'd poke me with his fingers, then use a stethoscope, and finally he'd ask me to get on the scale. Heart pounding, I'd put one foot and then the other on the cool gray slab. He'd push up the scale weights notch after notch, past 60, 70, 80, until finally the pointer stopped wobbling. He'd grimace; I'd cringe. He'd start talking in steel-laced sentences: "You've gained too much weight. It's just not pretty to be fat, not pretty at all. You don't want to walk around feeling ugly, now do you? None of the boys will like you. Look at Nancy [his daughter], how thin Nancy is. Why don't you be like her? You're too fat, Geneen, too fat. Fat is disgusting."

I'd stand there huddled around myself, shivering, facing him with bare budding breasts and thighs that were already too large. I'd try to think of other things while he talked—Ann's face, my dog wagging his tail—but sometimes a word of his would dip down into the heap into which I had folded myself and I'd shudder: Disgusting. Ugly. Fat. I'd think how next year I'd lose weight and then he'd like me; then he'd like me. He'd smile and tell me how pretty I was. I wanted him to smile and say something kind. Next year, maybe.

I look now at pictures of myself from those years—when I was eight to around fourteen or fifteen: me in a ballet recital wearing a blue tutu, me on the front lawn playing volleyball, me in my first formal dress—pink and glittering and wiremouthed. I looked like everyone else, with a body like most of the other girls. Not scrawny, not lanky, but certainly not fat.

When I was eleven, my mother told me I couldn't have two Good Humor ice creams in one day because I was getting fat. I was shocked and hurt, but I believed her. From that moment on, and for the next seventeen years, I blamed every one of my inadequacies on being fat.

My childhood journal, which I started the same year my

mother told me she was thinking about divorcing my father, speaks only fleetingly—once or twice in a period of three years—of worries about my parents. I remember dreaming about their divorce nightly, waking up screaming with fear and anxiety. Yet my journal chatters incessantly about my body; weighing ninety-two pounds instead of eighty-six; the size of my thighs, my ankles, my hips.

"I ate two frozen Milky Ways today," reads an entry dated 26 February 1963. "I snuck them up the stairs so Mom wouldn't see. I had a fight with her. She really gets on my nerves. I'll start a diet Monday. If I don't eat for two days, I can lose four pounds. Love ya, Geneen."

Food and feeling fat played a dual function: They allowed me to slip away from the pain of the present to a place where responsibility for the future was in my hands. My entire life began to focus on, to revolve around, food. My happiness became hinged on what I ate or didn't eat, instead of on situations I couldn't control: family distress, school problems, the rejection of a boyfriend or girlfriend.

When my mother's discontent was directed at me, I convinced myself that she didn't love me. Because she was, at the same time, critical of my body, I told myself her lack of love was because I was fat. The terrifying possibility of my parents' divorce got hooked up to my conviction that my mother didn't love me, which in turn seemed directly connected to my weight. I made myself—or, rather, my fat—responsible for my parents' unhappiness. I brought my fears to a level I could control—what went into and out of my mouth. Milky Ways hidden in my pajamas; Hostess Sno Balls stowed in a dresser drawer: these were my defense against slammed doors and raised voices. When I sensed a parental fight brewing, I would switch my awareness, as easily as you switch a TV channel, from feeling at the mercy of my mother and father to a world in which nothing existed but me and the sweetness on the roof of my mouth.

Eight years later, when I was nineteen, my parents were finally divorced. By that time I had eaten my way through junior high and high school, dieted my way through injections, coffee and cigarette fasts, and followed the advice of every new doctor from Los Angeles to New York who had written a book telling people how to eat.

Fat becomes your protection from anything you need protection from: men, women, sexuality (blossoming or developed), frightening feelings of any sort; it becomes your rebellion, your way of telling your parents, your lovers, the society around you, that you don't have to be who they want you to be. Fat becomes your way of talking. It says: I need help, go away, come closer, I can't, I won't, I'm angry, I'm sad. It becomes your vehicle for dealing with every problem you have.

If you take away the fat without uncovering the needs it is expressing, you are left without a way to say what you do or don't want to, or don't know how to, or feel you can't say directly. Fat speaks *for* you.

In our culture, it's unacceptable to be fat, which makes it seem self-destructive to continue to be overweight. Fat is regarded as a deviation from the norm; it is considered ugly, unfeminine, offensive, even disgusting. Fat sticks out; it is unavoidable, apparent. And it is precisely *because* it is a deviation, *because* it sticks out, *because* it is so devastating to be fat in a thin society, that it serves its function as communicator so well.

Eventually it gets so painful that you may be willing to listen to what your fat is saying. Like a baby who won't make its way down the birth canal until the womb becomes too small, your fat, though uncomfortable, is familiar and safe. There is something comforting about the discomfort—the familiarity of it—until suddenly the solace isn't there any longer. Until one day when the familiarity is not enough to keep you wrapped around yourself, and you are willing to move from what is known (fat and all its consequences) to what is not known (the needs it is fulfilling—and what being thinner permanently and all of *its* consequences are likely to be).

Listen closely. Speak to your fat and allow it to answer you. It may tell you that you were quite ingenious to sink yourself into its layers; that in doing so, you have enabled yourself to tolerate otherwise intolerable situations. Go back to the periods of your life in which you gained weight. Write a diet history. You will discover that as a child or a teen-ager or a confused adult, you didn't have the tools to express your inner needs and emotions. So you did what you could. You used what was around. You ate. When you come to understand that you were really taking care of yourself in the best way you knew how, you can release yourself from the stigma of "crazy" and "self-destructive." Acknowledge yourself for having discovered a way to survive. And once you acknowledge the needs your fat is expressing, you will begin to uncover ways to meet them other than eating. You will realize that being fat is not the mark of a glutton, or of someone out of control, but of someone who is in touch with her feelings. Fat is your attempt to *deal* with your feelings.

Look for a moment at the benefits of being fat. Visualizing yourself getting thinner and thinner, remember or imagine what it *feels* like to be thin—the clothes you are then able to wear, your dealings with people, how you handle your body. Take note that being thin isn't unequivocally wonderful, that there are frightening elements to that state, too: the pressure you may feel at being the center of attention; your uncertainty about handling the attractions of the opposite sex; ambivalence about your own sexuality.

I knew a woman named Anna. She came into one of my workshops absolutely determined to lose weight. She had tried everything—every diet published, every diet center established, every kind of traditional and/or quirky method to lose weight. She would lose it, then gain it back. In the group, she main-

tained with conviction that her fat had no purpose, that she
hated it and herself.

One evening, after a guided fantasy, she said, "I just realized that whenever I get thin, my husband Bob accuses me of
cheating." I asked her if that was true, if she did cheat.

"No," she said, "I really love him. I want our marriage to
work. But when I'm thin and we go to parties, if I even talk to
any other men, Bob makes a scene. He stomps out of the party,
takes a cab home and won't talk to me for days. I am so afraid
he'll leave me."

She told me she'd tried talking with him about it, asking him
if he would go with her for couple-counseling, but he refused.
Anna said, "He says there's nothing to talk about. He says it's
true that I cheat when I'm thin, period. I don't want to lose
him. I'll do anything to keep him."

Anything. Even get fat. And play the game of wanting to be
thin. That way, she could focus on herself and take the blame
for her inability to keep the weight off. She never looked at the
fact that in order to keep her marriage stable, she had to
endanger her health. And not allow herself the surge of power
and self-confidence she would receive from looking the way she
wants to look. When Anna felt best about herself, her husband
walked out. She was receiving the message that it is wrong to
look good, to feel good. More important than just sensing that
message, she had come to believe it.

If you had seen her in a supermarket, her hair in rollers,
buying *TV Guide*, two quarts of ice cream, potato chips, and
cookies, you'd have relegated her to the category of "helplessly
overweight, out of control, doesn't care about herself or her
marriage." How could she? What man would want to come
home to *that?*

When I looked, I saw a woman wrapping herself in layers of
fat with good purpose. I saw a woman directly in touch with
what she perceived as the bleak reality of her situation: that
she had to be fat in order to keep her husband. Anna ate

because it was the only way she knew how to hold onto what she believed she could not live without. She was trying to survive by holding onto what she loved.

Her situation, though more obvious than others, is not atypical. There are *always* good reasons why you eat in a seemingly chaotic and inexplicable manner. It often takes time, because of the cultural abhorrence of fat, to discover what these reasons are; but, if you are given time and awareness and support, they will make themselves known. Fat, although an effective solution to problems, is not usually a satisfactory one. You know, somewhere deep down you know, even while you are swallowing chunk after chunk of whatever you can find, that the food never quite gets to what is really bothering you. If the reason you eat is intangible—a need unexpressed, a desire unfulfilled, feelings unspoken—then no tangible substance is going to be able to meet it satisfactorily. Like trying to fit a star into the shape of a circle, there are always empty spaces; there is always a hunger that you can't define.

Look again at your feelings about fat and fat people. Chances are, they're myths.

The Loss of Ignorance

Once upon a time, I was beautiful.

My hair was thick and dark and glossy. My skin was smooth and soft as a ripe peach, unmarred by blemishes or wrinkles. My mouth was dark pink and my teeth white and even. My eyes were large and clear, a deep blue-green. Beautiful.

Unfortunately, I was four years old at the time. It's been downhill ever since.

Maybe my decline started when I broke my two front teeth during a race to the center of a Tootsie Pop. You know. How many licks does it take to get to the center? I cheated. I bit. Those two teeth came out long before my permanent ones were ready to come in. I smiled with my mouth closed for a long time. Cheaters never prosper.

There's a more likely origin to my fall from grace, though. As the eldest of three girls in a home where there was always plenty of food on the table and plenty of Ayds candies in the closet, I learned early how easy it is to get more when you're bigger than the other two people you're supposed to share with. I was the oldest; I got first crack at the cookies.

It works out. My youngest sister is "the thin one."

But I didn't really have any concept of myself as being different from anyone else. I honestly thought that as far as bodies went, mine was pretty much like everyone else's. If I had seen that for the delusion it was, would my life have been different? Might I be sitting here today in Jordache jeans (size 7)? I doubt it.

The terrible truth had to come from without. The tubbo is always the last to know.

One summer day my best friend Hildy and I lay on towels on the sidewalk in front of the stoop leading up to four garden apartments in Queens. Hildy lived upstairs to the left; I lived upstairs to the right. That made us inseparable, except in school, where it isn't so easy to bridge the gap between first and second grade. Hildy was a year older. I've always been attracted to those more worldly than I.

We were impatiently waiting to get tans. We turned every couple of minutes, too restless to stay still for long, and checking at each turn for any difference in color between the skin on our bellies and the skin under our bathing suits. Mine was a white two-piece with red polka dots and ruffles—the sort of suit any mother would be mortified to wear herself, yet would think nothing of putting on her daughter.

After a while, Shelly (who had moved into the apartment under Hildy's about a year before, and who was further distinguished by the fact that her father wasn't Jewish) came out and joined us. She also wore a two-piece bathing suit—but hers was a black bikini splashed with tropical flowers—the kind that most mothers wish they could get away with, and would never dream of putting on a kid. Shelly was my age, and she was more my friend than Hildy's.

Shelly's skin was darker than ours, and she tanned easily. We looked like two slices of Wonder White next to a slice of whole wheat. But even though I wished my tan were as dark as Shelly's, I didn't hold her personally responsible for the fact that it wasn't. I was a big-hearted kid.

The three of us passed some time rotating, checking, and wishing that our mothers would let us use suntan lotion. After a while we ran out of topics for immediate discussion and were quietly reflective for a few minutes. Hildy turned on her side and propped her head up on her hand. "You know, Sharon," she said, "Shelly looks a lot better than you do. You're *fat*."

If Jonathan had betrayed David, if Damon had betrayed Pythias, if Butch Cassidy had betrayed the Sundance Kid, their shock would not have been greater than mine. I was stunned—not only by the words, which were a thunderbolt from the blue, but by their source—Hildy, my best friend!

Of course, if I had been sixteen instead of six, I would have come back with some vile comment of my own concerning *Hildy's* figure. She wasn't exactly sylphlike herself. But I was six, and as I look back on it, Hildy's observation became a malevolent spirit, unleashed to haunt me forever.

I stood up with as much dignity as a stricken six-year-old in a white bathing suit with red polka dots and ruffles can muster, and went upstairs to our apartment, into my parents' room, and shut the door.

I climbed up on the bed so I could see my whole body in the big mirror over the dresser. Fat? Mommy and Daddy had never told me I was fat. Nobody had. I turned sideways. My stomach was round, like my face, and my thighs were pudgy. Hildy was right. It was true.

My parents had been in Weight Watchers early in the organization's existence. Even at that tender age, I knew that eating less food meant being less fat. Full of resolve, I then and there decided to go on a diet and stop being fat.

I had forgotten about it by dinnertime.

Many diets have come and gone since then. I weigh about sixty pounds less now than I did at my peak, but I'm still not even within nine points of a ten. I keep telling myself that if I can just be strong, if I can just be good, I can recapture the magic that was mine when I was four years old. Still, time is running out, and I often ponder the injustice that I am getting wrinkles before my skin has cleared up.

But the other day my friend Susan told me that she definitely would not, does not, think of me as being fat.

I've always been inclined to trust my friends.

—Sharon Sperling

Fat

Something you take in and just can't use. Fat hangs around reminding you of what wasn't totally digested, a layer of heavy water, something greasy.

Having so much, I used to dream that those tall, thin four-thirty shadows were really me. I pressed so hard it hurt, in punishment, squeezing myself into me, compressing what I didn't want. I spent afternoons with the shades drawn, examining and hating what I saw, longing for one of those svelte bodies dressed and undressed in *Vogue*. I used to set the scales back ten pounds. I still do.

When I was twelve I bought one of those Playtex rubber girdles (nobody knew), and only peeled it off with the door locked tight. Jessica's mother once said, "Lyn, you'll never get cold this winter, with fat legs like that." Now, how could something like fat, being only an extension of yourself, ever protect you from anything outside? Cells spreading, making you much more vulnerable. After all, fat people have many more places to bruise or to scar.

I sat in a room watching the river when the skinny girls were going across the state line, were necking in cars at Lake Bomoseen. I despised those layers I didn't need, hated the belly and hips that I squeezed into clothes at least one size too small. But what I hated most were my thighs, thighs that spread out on the bench at basketball practice. I used to lie on my back cycling air in my mother's gray living room until the room spun. White waves of the body. I was so ashamed I wouldn't even go to the beach. My mother always said, "Lyn, you're pretty: eat." And I curled into myself, eating M&M's in the brown chair, eating everything that made me worse, though I wanted to wear pleats and be thin.

In a furniture store in Rutland, Vermont, a man asked my mother, looking first at my sister, "Is it difficult having one daughter who's so lovely," and then he looked at me and added, "and then the other?" I hated my sister for being blond, her body like a Kean waif. I was jealous of her eggnogs and chocolate, of how meat had to be coaxed onto her bones.

Look, you can't camouflage anything or hold it in forever. It explodes. A rubber girdle pops—the elastic lets go. Then they know that there's more there than you can handle. Once when I was walking home from school the elastic on my underpants died. The next day somebody wrote "kike" on the blackboard. Both I knew were simply the result of fat. If you saw me now, you'd probably say, "but those thin wrists." These days, when I weigh over a hundred I break out in hives. But we all think of ourselves the way we were, especially when it comes to what we don't love.

I have never been good at getting rid of what I can't use. Old clothes or husbands. And when some man says love, I still don't believe him. So if I do wear my clothes too tight it's to remind myself (I still avoid every mirror, every plate-glass storefront) that my legs are not unlovable. I want you to see I finally am somebody you might just want to dance with. This me, waiting years underneath on the sidelines. It's been years of getting down to this. But it really is sweetest close to the bone.

—*Lyn Lifshin*

On Chubby Men

Another beer, and then he eyes the barmaid's legs and waist and thighs. "Needs to lose some weight," he grunts, "but just the same, I'd fuck her once." He orders pizza, buys a round, gains an appetizing pound.

—Patricia Monaghan

A Dialogue with Fat

Myself: Fat?

Fat: I'm listening.

Myself: I know this isn't a great way to begin trying for a new relationship, but I need to tell you something that I've been holding in for a while.

Fat: What is it?

Myself: I hate you.

Fat: (Silence)

Myself: I hate the way you crinkle around my legs and the way you fold my stomach in three parts when I bend over. I hate the way you keep me from getting into my size 6 and 8 and 10 clothes, the way you sag under my arms. I want you to go away and leave me alone forever.

Fat: But you've been hating me for quite a long time. I think it's time to consider something you have been overlooking: If you really wanted me to go away, I would be gone. *You* are the one who won't let *me* go. *I* have no investment in being here. All you have to do is want me to be gone and I will be.

Myself: Then why am I in so much pain because of you? Why would I hold onto something that causes me so much grief? I do, I really do, believe that if I were thin, my life would be better.

Fat: How?

Myself: I would have a lover; my nights would not be lonely; I wouldn't feel like such a blob, look like such a blob. I wouldn't be in such pain.

Fat: You're not in pain because of me. You're in pain because you're in pain . . . because there are nights when you want to be close to someone, when you want to hold someone, and there is no one there. You're in pain because when you wake up frightened at 3 A.M., you've got to deal with it alone. You've got to turn on the light, walk around your house, make a cup of tea. Alone. You get tired of the solitude, the silence; you want to curl up on someone's chest, have your hair stroked . . .

Myself: You're not telling me anything I haven't already discovered. I *know* I'm in pain because I feel so alone. That's why I started this conversation; that's exactly my point. It's because of you that I'm alone.

Fat: You have been wanting to be alone for years, and now, when you finally have the space, the only way you can feel all right about it is to gain twenty pounds and say that it's because of me that you are alone. You don't *want* a lover, and you're in pain because you think something is wrong with you because you don't; you're worried that you'll never want to live with anyone; you're worried that you'll die lonely.

Myself: Maybe.

Fat: You're still not willing to talk to me, are you?

Myself: Yeah, I am. It's just that it's difficult making friends with you, and so much simpler to hate you.

Fat: I understand; I really do. Now, why don't you talk more about your feeling that something is wrong with you because you are living alone and without a lover?

Myself: I don't take myself seriously. I believe that I am here to love someone, to provide nurturing and guidance, a warm body. I see myself as a receptacle, not as a source of anything. The only thing I have ever taken seriously has been my looks. I can remember being in about seventh grade and thinking that I would be extremely relieved to be married because then I could relax my eating habits; I wouldn't have to be concerned about my body anymore. I could stay in bed until eleven, watch soap operas and eat anything I wanted. I could get fat.

Fat: So the purpose of being thin was to catch a man?

Myself: Yes.

Fat: But now you don't have a man.

Myself: And I feel lost. I was never thin because I wanted to be thin; I was thin because I felt I needed to be in order to find the right husband. My life was geared to being beautiful in order to have a man occupy my life, validate me. Yet no relationship has been enough to make me happy for very long. Something in me remains unsatisfied and incomplete no matter how much in love I am. It always gets down to my wanting to break out and leave, to be alone . . .

Fat: Which is what you are doing now. Can you see that? Can you see that I am your protection? That I am your excuse not to do what you've been conditioned to do?

Myself: It's true—isn't it?—that no one expects a fat lady to
          find a husband. You give me space; you give me
          time. With you I can release myself from the bondage
          of the necessity to be flirtatious and sexy and on the
          hunt. You allow me relief from my own expectations.
          When I am thin, I think I have to have or to be
          pursuing a man. And I don't want to; I really don't
          want to. I want to develop my work; I've never given
          myself time to get to the bottom of that need for work
          and develop what I instinctively feel I am good at:
          writing and working with people. I need work so
          badly, and right now it seems as if I can't do both:
          have a relationship and explore the work situation,
          too.

Fat: That's because your work, until now, has been to be
          beautiful. If a man thought you beautiful, your work
          was done. You were a success. You could relax, put
          your energy into what he wanted from you that he
          could keep reflecting beauty back to you. You've
          never been willing to be alone for long enough to find
          out who you are when you're not trying to be someone
          else's vision. You're taking a big leap in choosing to
          be alone. You're doing something you've never done,
          and you're probably frightened about what's on the
          other side. It's no wonder you need protection. It's
          also no wonder that you're in a lot of pain right now.
          Just because you need to be alone doesn't mean that
          being alone is easy.

Myself: I get frightened a lot. The nights are hardest. I want
          to jump out of myself and land in someone's arms.
          But I feel so unattractive at this weight that I can't.

Fat: You can see how easy it is to blame me for your
          loneliness, then. You get to thinking that the pain is
          because you don't have a lover and that you don't
          have a lover because you're fat. This need for time

alone has been coming on for years, and most of you is ready to deal with it. But one part of you is kicking and screaming and using me to trick you into believing that it's because of me that you're up against yourself. Old parts of you, especially the fairy-tale voice that believes it needs a man to survive, hang on for dear life.

Myself: I don't like to admit this, but I can see that I've needed you in order to feel okay about not having a lover. I feel so ugly when I'm fat that I don't go running around half-naked, making eyes at the grocer or the gas station attendant. I stay inside myself because I feel no one could possibly want me.

Fat: It's important for you to know that you don't *have* to be fat in order to remain centered. With your conditioning, though, it's difficult for you to be thin and self-contained. Thin women, however, do find satisfying work; and some, no doubt, choose to be alone.

Myself: I imagine that's the next step: being thin *and* remaining centered.

Fat: Probably. But in the meantime it would be helpful to stop putting so much energy into hating me and start focusing on the reasons you created me to begin with.

Myself: After all this, I must say that it was quite ingenious to evolve such an effective buffer between me and what I perceive as cultural expectations of me . . . why are you laughing?

Fat: Because you started this conversation by telling me you hated me. And now you're congratulating yourself for creating me. Could it be that you like me?

Myself: I wouldn't go that far. But would you mind if I called you by another name? "Fat" is so—well, it's crude.

Fat: What do you have in mind?

Myself: How about "Pleasingly Plump"?

Fat: Forget it.

Her Funny Valentine

The dress store was just five doors nearer her building than the Barricini's. This was lucky, because if she faltered at the candy-store window and lost her will in the dark lumps of chocolate resting in their innocent pink and white frills, she could force herself a few steps further. There she'd be crisply recalled to responsible maturity by a calculating study of this season's clothes and the ideal forms that didn't quite fill them.

Mornings weren't so dangerous. Today, for instance, she had awakened to the alarm at seven, staggered across the room to reset it for seven-thirty, and curled comfortably back under the blankets to finish her dreams. The seven-thirty alarm disguised itself as the shrieking climax of a cops-and-robbers drama she'd seen the night before on TV and whose dream version she preferred now, with herself doubling as chief mobster and luscious moll. She awoke at eight, just in time to be exactly fifteen minutes late, if she hurried.

She hesitated painfully over which maternity blouse to stuff herself into for the day. She'd lost twenty pounds over the last three weeks, and thought she was almost ready for red, but the longer she stared into the mirror, the more hugely all the remaining pounds bulged back at her. So it was brown again, just when she was starting to feel daring, probably as a hangover from last night's dreams.

No time for exercises this morning, or any other morning so far this week. She'd had to make them up every evening before dinner, dizzy and weak from the proud hunger she could never accept as routine. Today she'd have to skip breakfast as well, in violation of all diet rules; but with Angie's wedding so close, and with it her first minor victory, she felt reckless and ready to face an empty-bellied morning at the store.

The subway would have turned her stomach anyway. She was beginning to realize that everyone had trouble squeezing through the crowd around the door, and when she sat down in the space left by a normal-sized businessman, she had only to sit up very straight with her arms closely crooked over her handbag to fit in pretty well. The people on either side of her didn't even glare once at her hips, usually the most offending part of her bulk.

As she waited at Chock Full o' Nuts for her morning coffee, she felt no temptation to buy a corn muffin. In fact, the thought of butter oozing softly into the yellow surface crumbs was slightly revolting, a recalling of something greasy and weak in her former appetites. Armed by her hunger, she faced the time clock defiantly and punched in at nine-sixteen, not caring that she'd be docked a quarter-hour's pay. She made her entrance to the Basement Housewares selling floor wearing a tough little smile, daring anyone to accuse her of lateness.

"Glad you're here, Elaine," the floor manager substituted, she was sure, for something more critical. "There's a new shipment of Pyrex, and the girls'll have to help shelve. You okay alone at the register?"

Of course she could handle the cash register alone. Hairy little hippie, she thought; he gets one promotion and thinks everyone else is a trainee imbecile. She watched Larry slouch over to one of the salesgirls, a blond nitwit named Charmaine, of all pretentious things.

None of the salesgirls had any sense. They'd let that fool Larry paw them all over; they climbed up on ladders like stockboys, leaving their legs defenseless against his absent-minded caresses. Maybe they liked it, though: thought it gave them an in with the boss. If he ever tried that stuff on her, he'd get a space shoe in his face. Maybe that's what caused him to keep his distance from her, made him show a decent respect for her age. Elaine looked down past her bulges, where three weeks of starvation were revealing her feet, like the moon's slow return from eclipse. Maybe it wasn't respect he showed after all. She could face the fact now, when her prison of fat was finally giving way.

The morning picked up as customers accumulated. They'd dawdle around for an hour, up and down the aisles of cheap dishcloths and teakettles, and then irritably crowd her checkout counter, impatient at having to wait another five minutes. She was glad when Charmaine relieved her for lunch; her feet were swelling, and the dizziness had set in early.

It took a while to find her yogurt in the employee refrigerator. She liked the way her lunches were occupying a smaller and smaller part of the shelf; it made her think she could get smaller, too. Of course, the little carton wasn't very filling, but she was getting to like its unsatisfying taste: half comforting custard, half tart sour cream. She told herself it was lunch and dessert in one.

"Still dieting, dear?" That was scrawny Edith, from Notions, who always knew how to annoy her. "Better watch out; you'll get yourself sick that way. Nothing really does it like good eating habits, my husband always said. He had more patients who went on these crazy fads of yours till they collapsed, and then they just put it right back on. And you don't look at all well lately."

Elaine seethed as she watched Edith chew her spare

little chicken sandwich. Some women thought because they'd been married to doctors once, that made them better than you. But face it, she thought; we're two old bags in the same boat now, getting old fast in a five-and-dime store's employee lunchroom, and I'm just a little more inflated a bag than you are.

"I'm not dieting," she protested aloud. "It's just my niece's wedding. Angie's after me all the time with fittings and rehearsals till I don't have a minute to breathe. I just forget to eat these days."

"Well, I can understand that you want to look nice for the wedding, but really, you shouldn't overdo it."

Elaine crushed her yogurt carton, exasperated, and left for Housewares in a bad mood that the afternoon made even worse. Two different customers tried to con her into giving them discounts on pots they'd dented themselves, and Larry fell for their lies, probably just to embarrass her. And she had four overrings during the closing rush because Charmaine kept mumbling the wrong prices to her. Her train stalled on the way home, and she had to stand for half an hour in the worst possible crush, with wet raincoats dripping all over her and people's damp, smelly bodies making her sick to her stomach. Just when she was ready to faint, she reached her stop, in time to collapse on a bench, where she sat and watched bright squiggles of light dance on the sooty tracks until her strength returned.

Outside, the fresh February rain revived her. Under her striped umbrella she was an unjostled island. Elaine sloshed home slowly, hypnotized by the gleaming streetlights reflected in the dark puddles. At the red-lit sidewalk in front of Barricini's she stopped for her nightly test of strength. There, draped in thick red velvet at the center of the window, lay a deep heart-shaped box of the most beautiful chocolates she'd ever seen. The swirls on top followed each one's varied outlines, and sprinkled surfaces of powdered nuts and sugars alternated with glittering gold and silver foils and subtle dark spheres. She was about to imagine how it would feel to unwrap and bite into one of the golden ones when a stubborn portion of her mind snapped out an image of herself, a huge middle-aged woman drooling over a box of candy meant as a lover's Valentine. She tilted her umbrella to shade her eyes from the warm red light and headed for Loretta's Clothing and Accessories, where her dress was waiting. She'd tried it on every Friday since she'd started her diet, and it made all her hunger pangs worthwhile. Tonight it fit her just a little short of perfectly, and by next Saturday, if she gave up breakfast entirely, she could appear at the wedding as a ripe beauty of an aunt. The dress was an oversized woman's dream: loose where she was loose, but billowing kindly into a generous exaggeration of the classic hourglass shape. All she needed now was a waistline, and her sister and her sister's stuck-up daughter would be sorry they'd almost talked her out of attending the wedding. The photographers would want her in all the pictures; none of this nonsense of not being able to fit her left side into the frame: she'd be the best-dressed woman there.

She drifted home, through the Wilsons' living room and up the stairs to her rented room in a haze of anticipated glamour. When she first looked at the bed, she thought a rejected daydream had crept into her chosen fantasy: a devil's predinner delusion.

But it was real. The shabby bedspread kept its heart-shaped imprint even after she dreamily lifted the perfect chocolate box. No one sent Valentine's Day presents to fat old Housewares cashiers. Then she realized, with furious shame, that it was all a joke. Someone, either Larry or the salesgirls or Edith with her chicken sand-

wiches and scrawny chicken-yellow arms; or maybe one
of the Wilsons or even Angie . . . someone had noticed
that she was starving herself, trying to become a normal
thin person, and had hated her enough to plant this in
her room.

Elaine shook the chocolates wildly into the wastebasket.
The top layer rattled out, but she had to fumble clumsily
at the greasy paper to get at the others. The last candy
got caught in the V of the heart and crushed open under
her thumb as she pushed it after the rest. Automatically
her thumb went to her mouth; and as she licked off the
cherry cordial, all the sweet tastes she'd fought off in the
past weeks came rushing back. She remembered her
morning Danishes, and the little sweet cupcakes she'd
eaten on her afternoon break. Then, more bitter, there
were all the diets she'd failed at; the years of stepping on
and off scales that surely were broken; and the first time
her parents had tried to trick her into thinness by telling
the other girls' mothers that she was allergic to chocolate,
so that she sat through endless birthday parties with a
dish of plain vanilla ice cream, watching skinny girls
gobble all the cake. And now she was old, forever fat;
and the world wanted her to stay that way.

From a blind, blank, hurting cave she groped, all hunting fingers, in the trash, fishing out the pretty chocolates,
chewing and swallowing them, wastebasket fuzz and all.
When the last one was gone, she lay heavily on the
sagging bed, listening sickly to the voices rising from the
Wilsons' kitchen.

"What do you mean, you brought me candy? I never
saw any candy. You could at least get your wife a card
on Valentine's Day."

"I'll go up right now and show you. I left them right in
Elaine's room when I came in. I just wanted to surprise
you—"

"You left them in that pig's room? Why didn't you just feed them to the dog? At least he'd have the sense to stop eating them when he got sick and there'd be a couple left for me."

Elaine covered her head with a pillow and squeezed her eyes shut. They wouldn't come in now if she was asleep; she knew her rights as a tenant. And they wouldn't get away with calling her a pig, either. They'd have to go to bed sometime, and then she'd show them what a real pig could do. They'd have to hunt for their breakfast tomorrow, all right. She'd eat everything in sight and pack herself a hero sandwich for lunch, maybe even a coffee cake. And at the wedding, she'd show them how embarrassing a fat aunt could really be. She wasn't going to tuck any wedding cake under her pillow waiting for some fat-loving Prince Charming pervert to come along. She'd eat it right there in front of them all, in her old black funeral sack, wearing all her rhinoceros folds of flesh intact. Elaine burrowed deep under the heavy blankets and dreamed of queasy feasts.

—Linda Ostreicher

Lists*

If I were thin, men would . . .
 love me
 annoy me
 buy me a sports car
 want my body
 not leave me alone
 not know I needed them

 take it as an invitation
 hurt me
 pay
 be overwhelmed by me
 have to book me months
  in advance

If I were thin, women would . . .
 want my old clothes
 try to feed me
 ask who my diet doctor
  is
 assume I was fooling
  around
 wonder when I was
  gonna get fat again

 include me
 respect me
 think I had no
  compassion
 watch how I ate

 be threatened

If I were thin, I would . . .
 be sexual
 wear a bikini
 be more willing to get up
  in the morning
 get everything

 wear shorts
 be frightened
 feel unprotected

 be more self-conscious

*A compilation from the members of the Breaking Free workshops.

leave the lights on more often

be less self-conscious

feel there is nothing I couldn't do

be outrageous

If I ate whatever I wanted, I would . . .

have acne

be overwhelmed with guilt

be poor

have lots of cavities

eat doughnuts

be satisfied

not feel any better

be fat

be happy

be normal

Being fat means I can't . . .

get my picture taken

wear designer jeans

run upstairs

get good service in stores

be a ballerina

be sexual

be seen in public buying cookies

relax

accept praise

relate to people without feeling apologetic

If I were as thin as I wanted, I couldn't . . .

be alone

eat

have needs

be powerful

say no to anyone

have a good excuse to say no to sex

stay thin

protect myself

cry

be asexual

Being fat means I can . . .

settle for less

feel numb

make excuses

hate myself

not threaten other women

survive in a famine

be rebellious

always have a goal

keep my mother happy by making her miserable

not fit in

eat

A woman is supposed to . . .

smell good

be like the "Oil of Olay" woman

be last

be a whore in the bedroom

be a lady in the living room

know her place

always be willing

be all things to all people

be coy without being aggressive

be cute, sexy, nonscientific

be thin and attractive at all times

support her man

be helpless

be helpful

eat the burned one

lose

A woman is not supposed to . . .

scream

sweat

take care of her own car

complain

be hairy

like sex too much

be fat, ugly, muscular, smart

be serious, selfish, competent, independent

Thin women are . . .

bitchy and cold

lucky

manipulative

happy

not lonely   coveted
only liked for their looks
everything I'm not

Fat women are . . .
   kind and caring   miserable
   warm   sneaky eaters
   jolly   happy
   supportive   good lovers

Apple Cheeks and Thunder Thighs

"You're all circles," my friend Mark said to me in high school. "There's no point in losing weight. When you get skinny you just look like a set of deflated circles, and that looks silly." I glared at him. I sulked. It didn't help. "Look, Geneen," he said, trying another approach, "you have beautiful hair and a clear complexion. That's good enough. Why don't you just give up this ridiculous dieting and accept the fact that your body is round? So what?"

"So *what?*" I screeched. "It's ugly—*that's* what. Never! I will never accept this body until it's thin. Never."

Mark, who was six feet two and a half, wiry, and a guiltless Oreo cookie lover, could not understand what it meant to be round. When he looked at me he saw my hair, my eyes, my skin, the general shape of my body. When *I* looked, I saw legs like tree trunks and a face like the moon's. Nothing else. I saw nothing but fat.

And how I hated that word. Ever since Sidney Schulman chased me in the school yard when I was eight, taunting me with "Moon Face, Moon Face, Fat Face, Fat Face," I had cringed at the word "fat." I wished later I had called back at him, "Frog Eyes, Frog Eyes, Croak, Croak," but it didn't occur to me then. By the time I was twelve, my body image had jelled into a mold shaped by other people's opinions: my mother's ("Apple Cheeks," "Chubby") my brother's ("Thunder Thighs"), Sidney Schulman's (see above), the family doctor's ("fat" is "ugly").

Then, in the ninth grade, Richard Pepper came onto the scene. He sat behind me in homeroom. I was the new girl in school and a perfect target for abuse. Every time I turned around in my seat, he'd puff out his cheeks like a squirrel with nuts in its mouth and look at me with mocking eyes. As the leader of the bullies, he got all his friends to do it too, so within a week there was a creepy boy puffing up his cheeks in each of my classes, in the halls between classes, in town after school. My reaction to the squirrel faces was the same each time—when I saw the puff, I'd turn away, humiliated, pretending nothing had happened. On one particularly devastating day, when I was leaving a friend's house, I saw Richard walking on the same street. When he saw me he crossed to the same side as I, and with a smirk on his face and puffs in his cheeks he grabbed my breasts, squeezing them very hard as he passed me. I stood there, limp and passive. He knew I was too humiliated to fight back. He knew I was afraid of him and that I believed myself to be the space-face he gleefully tortured. He knew I'd do anything for him to like me, even let him molest me.

When I was a sophomore, the boys in the senior class made up names for each of us girls. The names were a secret; they called us by coded initials. My name was "P.F.C." A year later I found it meant "Pregnant-Faced Cow." Shocked at the cruelty, I was nevertheless convinced of its truth. Even now, sixteen years later, it is painful to recall, so painful that this is the first time I have talked about it.

Moon Face; Thunder Thighs; Pregnant-Faced Cow—I could trace the origins of my body image to the names I was called. I willingly gave a slice of my soul to each one of the people who were cruel to me, and then convinced myself that I needed their approval in order to be whole.

What astounds me now is that I never, not once, thought to question the validity of any of those names. If Mark thought my body was a bunch of circles, deflated or not, so it was. My brother called me "Thunder Thighs" because it was true; I had thunder thighs. Richard Pepper made fun of my face because it did, it really did, look like a nut-loaded squirrel's.

For years I dreamed about being thin. I wanted to step out of my body and grow a new one: lithe, graceful and thin; very, very thin. Eventually I did. I became anorectic and shrank to ninety pounds; yet when I looked in the mirror, I still saw thunder thighs and a moon face. I saw Robert Pepper's smirk; heard Mark's voice: circles upon circles upon circles. Thinner and thinner until my face was drawn and cavernous, my breasts the size of mosquito bites. And still the mirror showed fat, mounds and mounds of fat.

In my workshops I ask the members to walk up to the mirror and describe what they see.

Woman #1 approaches the mirror slowly, hesitantly. She is about five feet four and weighs one hundred twenty-five pounds. "I haven't looked in a full-length mirror in two years," she says. "This is very difficult."

"What do you see?" I ask.

"I see hair that's messy, skin that's broken out, fat arms, no waist, big boobs, fat legs."

"Anything else?"

"Well, I like my eyes. They're nice."

I ask her to turn and face the rest of the group.

"What do you see," I ask the others, "when you look at her?"

"Beautiful hair, a very sweet face."

"No fat at all. You have a well-proportioned body; it curves in all the right places."

"I don't see any overweight. I like your eyes, too. There's something about you that's tremendously appealing—you're vivacious."

"If I were a man, I would want to go out with you."

The group continues with their observations. No one mentions fat; yet that is all Woman #1 sees.

Woman #2 volunteers to go next. She is about five feet five and weighs one hundred ninety. Before she has a chance to look in the mirror, she says, "I feel trapped in this body. I hate it."

"But the mirror—look at yourself in the mirror. What do you see?" I ask.

"I see a fat face, no neck, a double chin, sagging arms, mammoth legs. There's no shape at all to my body. I see a person enclosed in inner tubes."

"Is there any part of your body that you like?"

"You mean just out and out *like?*"

"Yes," I answer.

She looks at me somberly. "No."

She faces the group; it's time for their feedback. She holds her breath, clenches her fists.

Woman #2 is unmistakably fat, and no one tells her she isn't. They talk to her about her face, her hair, their feelings when they are around her:

"You carry your weight well, as if you are not afraid."

"A twinkly face. I like looking at you."

One person tells her that she is inspired by her courage: "When I first met you, you seemed so 'out there' with your problems that it frightened me. But over the last few weeks, your honesty and willingness to examine your problems have opened the way for me to do the same. Thank you."

Woman #2 is visibly moved. Her hands hang loosely by her sides. She sits down.

Woman #3 walks up to the mirror. She is five feet three and weighs one hundred five pounds. She fidgets, wrings her hands, finally moves toward the mirror.

"Sometimes I like my face," she says, "because when I smile it makes me feel better. But my body . . . well, actually, my arms are okay, because I hammer nails all day—they are muscular, and I like that. But my waist and my thighs—they waddle and shake. I feel very self-conscious when I walk down the street. I need to lose about ten or fifteen pounds. Fifteen would be better, but ten would be okay."

She turns to the group and they speak:

"Perfect body. I would sell my mother for your legs. *She* would sell herself to *give* me those legs."

"You're gorgeous. And so kind. If I were lost and saw you on the street, I would ask you for help."

"Graceful and funny and beautiful. Looking at you makes me feel good."

She tries to protest; I ask her to be silent and hear what is being said. When the feedback is finished, I ask her what she has heard.

"Well," she says, "I heard that I wasn't *that* big."

"Is that all you heard?"

"That's all I believed." She sits back down.

I have never met a woman who liked her body. Weight has little to do with it, although it often seems as if fat is the problem: "If only I were thin, I'd be happy. I'd like myself; everything would be all right." But if fat is truly the problem, why do thin women hate their bodies as much as their heavier counterparts do? Why do thin women insist on seeing fat where there is none?

Your body is your statement, as a woman, to the world.

People often judge your intelligence, competence, and creativity by the way you look. You are defined and you define yourself according to how you see your body. Body image, then, becomes a complex issue.

Part of the process of unconvoluting your body image is realizing that your intrinsic value as a human being is *not related* to your extrinsic body weight, regardless of what the media tells you. You can be fat *and* sensitive, creative and competent. Fat has nothing to do with intelligence or vitality; beauty and fat are not mutually exclusive.

Many of us forget that the abilities to give and receive love, to compromise, to listen, the qualities upon which our lives depend, *do not weigh a pound*.

Another step in seeing your body clearly is developing the awareness that you are not in the present with yourself, that your ability to see your body without distortion has been plowed under by voices from the past. As long as there is childhood, there will be a Sidney Schulman, a Richard Pepper, and well-meaning families. But that's no reason to carry their taunts around with you for the rest of your life; no reason to continue internalizing their voices so that they become your own. The hardest thing to believe is that when you look in a mirror, you are *not* seeing what is actually there. That is never more apparent than when a thin woman walks up to the mirror and exclaims that she is fat. Even when a fat woman describes herself, what she sees is invariably worse than what is actually there.

Can a woman hate her body and still love herself?

Look at your own body—really look at it. Where does it curve? What is the texture of your skin? Try to observe with objectivity. If you came upon yourself in a painting by Matisse you would probably think yourself lovely. Looking at yourself with an artist's eye, what might you see? Anything that can release you from the harshly distorted view with which you have been judging your hips, thighs, arms, will help you. Stay in the present. The first step in developing a positive body image is accepting the body you have. You might as well accept it: you walk around in it every day, and so far, your rejection of it hasn't changed it. Acceptance means being able to look at your body without disgust. It also means disassociating fat from ugly or unlovable and reminding yourself that your body is only one aspect of you.

Look at yourself in the mirror for at least five minutes a day. When a negative judgment arises, replace it with a positive observation. Touch yourself in those areas you find unacceptable. Soothe them. This is *your* body—it's carried you through some pretty rough times. Love it a little. Love it a lot.

Nothing, no one responds to rejection—not a child, not your body. You have been filled with loathing at the sight of your arms, neck, face for years—and it hasn't helped. So you have stopped looking in mirrors, and you won't let even your lover or spouse touch you in the places you find repulsive. *You* don't want to accept your body, either. You are afraid that if you do, it will never change. So you continue to cringe at the sight of your own flesh. You grow old wishing you had someone else's body.

Rejection and disgust do not, however, lead to change. If they did, you would have long since given yourself a different body.

Acceptance does not lead to indolence or complacency. Awareness is a partner of acceptance. Once you become fully aware of what you are doing, you are able to make a decision about whether you want to keep on doing it. If, for instance, you tell yourself you can't eat ice cream and then go ahead and eat it anyway, only to feel guilty afterwards, you will never observe how ice cream feels in your stomach. Do you like the coldness? Does it give you a stomachache? If eating ice cream puts you in pain and you are quiet enough to hear that, you can then decide not to eat a gallon of it at a sitting—not because you *can't* but because you don't feel well when you do. Once you become fully aware of the effects of what you are doing without the need to beat yourself up about it, it becomes easier to give up doing something that actually causes you discomfort. Ironically, it is by doing what you are most afraid of—accepting yourself as you are now—that you will get to where you want to be, that you will change. Change is a natural result of awareness.

How do you know where acceptance will take you if you've never allowed yourself to feel it?

I am in high school again and I am leaving my friend's house to walk home. The squirrel king, Richard Pepper, is walking on the same street, and when he sees me he crosses to my side. With a smirk on his face and puffs in his cheeks, he nips my breast. I act quickly—I grab his balls and squeeze them hard. He winces, tries to loosen my grasp. It remains firm. Looking him straight in the eye, I say, "Don't you ever squirrel your cheeks at me again, mister. Same with your friends. Because next time, I won't let these go, and you'll have to get a job somewhere as a court eunuch." He manages to squeak out a surrender. I tighten my grasp one more time so that he knows I'm serious. Richard Pepper limps home.

Dieting: Always on Mondays

The first one was a normal one (I was eleven): cutting down on bread, potatoes and sweets, eating fruit between meals. I lost weight, felt better about myself. The second one (I was thirteen) was a variation thereof with a few quirks: meatballs with raisins on Wednesdays, prunes and roast beef for dinner on Saturday and Tuesday. By sixteen, I had become a fanatic.

I am fifteen. My mother picks me up at the bus station; it is the end of the summer, and I have just spent eight weeks at camp, linking braces with Mark Gold and not giving a thought to the ropes and ropes of licorice from the canteen that I ate every day. I am in love; my mother says I am fat. She says that she herself is also fat and so is my cousin Laura. My mother makes phone calls. Two days later the three of us are standing in front of a doctor who claims he can help us lose weight. He weighs us, takes our blood pressure, listens to our beating hearts, and injects something into our arms with what sounds like a staple gun. We don't ask him what's in the shot. We are mute, passive, obedient. He tells us in a German accent not to eat between meals. "Even if you eat a hot fudge sundae," he says, "do it at the end of a meal. Never, never anything in between."

He sends us to the front desk. A plump nurse named Cathy with purple eyelids and a scarlet mouth is seated in front of a row of Tupperware containers, each filled with a different size and color of pill. To her right is a phone, to her left a typewriter. I am dazed by the sight; I count the containers—sixteen in all. Such lovely colors. I like the emerald green best. One at a time we walk up to the desk. She looks at the chart the doctor has made out, takes out a small white envelope, and counts fourteen pills, two a day for a week. She gives my mother yellow ones, Laura white ones, and me, passion-pink pills. She charges my mother $50 for each of us to see the doctor and $7 per week's supply. Wishing us luck, she smiles sweetly and walks us to the door. We leave, clutching our envelopes. I have no idea what is in the pills or how they work. I ask no questions. All I want is to lose weight. "It's magic," I tell my friend Lizzy a week later. "I've lost six pounds!" Lizzy, wanting some magic of her own, uses her allowance that she's been saving for three months and pays a visit to the doctor and the plump nurse.

Lizzy and I compare notes daily. I settle on a diet of no breakfast, Grape-Nuts for lunch, and half a cup of applesauce for dinner. Lizzy prefers one hot fudge sundae a day. We both take the pills religiously. We continue to lose weight. Seventeen pounds and two months later I am still taking the pills, but no more weight is coming off. I complain to Cathy, the nurse, whom I see weekly; the doctor seems to be either out of town or in business meetings. I don't miss him. Cathy upgrades me to the next level of pills—the emerald-green lovelies.

But something is happening that I don't understand. I am edgy and tense; I can't sleep at night. Same with Lizzy. And now with Rebecca, with whom Lizzy has shared the magic. Having our own phones, we spend the hours from midnight to dawn whispering complaints about our bodies. We think the nervousness could be from the pills, but we don't know; besides, we don't want to risk the possibility of going off them. They have become our gateway to thinness and therefore to our happiness.

If a week goes by and we haven't lost weight, we rope my brother, three years my junior, into buying our pills. We don't want to see Cathy and get weighed, so we tell Howard that we need to buy some medicine; could he please get it for us? We drive to the office, write down what we need on a slip of paper and hand it to him. We wait in the parking lot. Every time he comes out he says, "What is that place? Some kind of diet doctor's office? I've never seen so many pills. Where's the doctor? Why is the nurse so fat?" We shush him with ice cream, tell him to stop asking so many questions. We are safe for another week.

I go through high school on green pills, never losing another pound but terrified to stop for fear I might gain weight. My mother, ignorant of what an amphetamine is, continues to take the pills as well, though less frequently than I.

I am a speed freak and I don't even know it.

In college I call Cathy long distance. I send her a check; she sends me the pills. She thinks maybe I should upgrade my dose in order to lose more weight. (I am not fat, but I think I am huge.) So I graduate to big red capsules.

I am nineteen. I hide the pills from my roommate, from my boyfriend. My boyfriend finds them in my purse one day, asks me what they are. When I tell him, he is horrified. "How long?" he asks. "Since I was fifteen." He is more than horrified; he is frightened about my health. He tells me about amphetamines and what they do to your body. He begs me, pleads with me to stop taking them. Every time he finds one, he flushes it down the toilet. He tells my roommate. They flush in harmony. I am secretly relieved. I want help but I don't know what for. Eventually—I can't remember how—I stop.

But it is only to go on to the next diet and the next. Protein with ketchup for breakfast, lunch and dinner; two bananas a day; the mistake of fried chicken for every meal. Stillman's, Atkins, Weight Watchers, until I become a vegetarian and food-combining expert. I stop the intake of all protein; I eat only raw food. I fast on water for days at a stretch. I become anorectic and drop to ninety-two pounds: my friends call me "Bones."

Within a year I am up to a hundred forty-five pounds. I am twenty-seven. In the past twelve years I have gained and lost over five hundred pounds. The absurd thing is that even at my heaviest, I was never fat. Chunky, yes. Plump, yes. Fat, no.

Fat is taking up two seats on the bus; fat is having to shop at "Pretty and Plump" for your clothes; fat is having to go through a doorway sideways. But to American women, fat is what insurance company charts say it is; fat is what a model isn't. Fat is five pounds more than scrawny. Fat has become the national obsession; it is a curse. Fat is the symbol for anything you are that you don't want to be. Fat has nothing to do with how much you weigh.

But it's difficult to see it like that. You look in the mirror and you see cellulite and sagging arms. You're getting old; you're not measuring up. You decide to fix it, fix yourself. The

American-woman cure-all: The Diet. Being thin means being happy. You decide to go on a diet. Having many to choose from (a different one in each magazine), you decide on one that doesn't look too hard. After ten days you've lost a few pounds, maybe more than a few. But then the unforeseen happens: an unexpected phone call or visitor, an invitation to dinner, and the spell is broken.

You're off on a binge. Everything the diet doesn't allow: peanut butter and marshmallows, ice cream, cookies. What's the *matter* with you? Why can't you stay on a diet? You tell yourself that you're disgusting, nothing but a mass of fat; no willpower. You make another resolve: Tomorrow; I'll diet tomorrow. In anticipation you eat a half gallon of ice cream before you go to sleep, to seal the pact. Now you *have* to diet. And you *do* . . . until the next binge.

So why can't you stay on a diet?

Because diets are not made to stay on.

Because diets are humiliating. Because they are built on deprivation. Because they teach you that you cannot be trusted. Because they usurp your private, personal power: that of deciding what you will put into your own mouth, your own body. Because when you let someone else—be it a deceased doctor in New York, a live one in California, an organization, or the author of a printed article—tell you what should feel right inside you, something in you, something you have no control over, rebels, stands up for itself, and says, "No way. This is my body."

When you go on a diet, you relinquish the responsibility of learning how to nourish yourself. And sooner or later it backfires, and you binge.

A binge is the other side of a diet; it is built into it; it is inevitable. For every diet there is an equal and opposite binge. Maybe not now, but in a week. And if not in a week, then in a month or six months. Bingeing is *part* of dieting. The pendulum swings to the other side in an attempt to get you back to the middle.

Where and what is that middle? Moderation? What *is* that? It's not thinking about dinner at breakfast or breakfast at dinner. It's going out to eat with friends and ordering what appeals to you, even if it is fettucine with cream sauce— instead of ordering cottage cheese with canned pineapple slices on a leaf of lettuce and then going home and eating the contents of the refrigerator when you are alone.

When you eat in the "middle," you eat in the present moment. You listen to your body. You trust the messages it gives you. You don't eat because it is breakfasttime or lunch-time or dinnertime; you realize there is no pattern to your hunger. You probably can't remember the last time you felt hungry; you probably think of hunger as a frightening experience.

Diets don't work. If they did, binges would not exist.

Diets *can't* work. They create in you the desire for what you can't have. If you weren't obsessed with food before you dieted, you are by the time you finish.

So many women I see only know how to diet or to binge. When I tell them to eat what they want, to forget about dieting, they look at me as if I were crazy. "You've got to be kidding, Geneen—if I do that I'll blow up like a blimp. I'll eat everything in sight. I'll eat twenty-four hours a day." They think because I tell them to eat what they want that I am telling them to binge. They are so used to depriving themselves that eating what they want sounds alien, frightening.

Think of the distortion of that. Think how much mistrust and fear it must take for you to say, "No, I can't give myself what I want. I *must* deprive myself. Deprivation is the only way. I am so wild that if I let myself loose, I will trample everything." What a tenuous way to live, feeling that you have a monster inside. That you must cage it, that it might escape at any moment. Diets give you the message that at your core you are untrustworthy, wild. At your core you are bad.

When you finally do it, when you let yourself eat what you want and stay with yourself while you are doing it, it takes a while for you to realize that if you listen to your body, it will not lie. It will tell you exactly what to eat and when. It will tell you when to stop. You might have to eat chocolate chip cookies for two weeks, one cooked batch and one raw batch. Or go to the store and buy the Sara Lee brownies you have been wanting and not eating for ten years. You might have to eat at strange hours of the day; you might seem a little eccentric to your friends. You might have to gain some weight. But eventually you will lose weight. And you will maintain the weight that is best for your body without a struggle.

The body responds to trust, to ease. When you are no longer depriving it by dieting, there is no push to devour everything but the dining room table. Food becomes your friend; you start using it as a way to satisfy a physical need. *You* become your friend. You start discovering other ways to satisfy nonphysical needs. Just as you wouldn't think about going to the bathroom when you don't have to, you won't think about eating if you are not hungry.

A woman came into one of my workshops four weeks ago. She introduced herself the first night as a drug addict, an alcoholic and a compulsive eater. She said she'd never been able to control herself. "I've been like this for twenty years. Look at me; it's disgusting. I've been to A.A., O.A., drug rehabilitation programs, Weight Watchers. You name it." Her voice shaking, she started to cry.

When I told the group, at the end of that first night, to spend the week eating what they wanted when they were hungry and to stop when they were full, she looked at me and said, "I can't. I can't do that. I'll go crazy if I do." I told her I didn't believe her. I told her that if she could unlearn everything she had learned about herself—that she had no willpower; that she couldn't be trusted; that, left to her own devices, she would destroy herself—she would find a woman/child starving for the chance to prove her ability to nurture herself. She stared at me, dazed, unbelieving.

Last night she walked into the group smiling. "Something is happening," she said. "I can't really explain it, but it seems like I'm getting a taste of freedom. It's not that I haven't eaten a lot this week, because I have; it's just that sometimes I'm not eating frantically, and I even left some food on my plate when my husband and I went out to eat the other night. I haven't done that since I was eight." She was silent for a minute or so, then turned to me and said, "I'm fifty-six, and I feel like a flower about to blossom."

If I told you you didn't have to be obsessed with food; if I said, "No matter how many times you have gained and lost weight for no matter how many years, you can learn to listen to your body; you can eat whatever you want; you can reach a comfortable weight and never have to go on another diet again," would you believe me? Would you dare?

My mother wrote in a recent letter that she had driven past the diet doctor's office and it looked as if it had been gutted by a fire. I wasn't sorry. I knew I should have been, but I wasn't. Maybe someone swallowed sixteen containers of rainbow pills and exploded like a bomb into streaks carrying the colors of the pills. The green lovelies must have created quite a spectacle. I can't help wondering, though, whatever happened to Cathy, the purple-eye-shadowed, scarlet-mouthed nurse. I'll bet she reformed. I'll bet she went natural, wiped off her makeup, and is sitting in some burgundy living room with lace curtains and lots of pillows, telling people to forget about diets and start listening to their bodies. With her background, she'd be great. People would listen. If you see her, say hello.

Cookies

It's thirty years ago, and I am breaking my first diet. I see myself walking up Nostrand Avenue on my way home from junior high school. I have spent my carfare on sweets, so I am hurrying, trying to jog along nearly as fast as a bus. At the same time, I am stuffing candy in my mouth, feeling guilty and driven as well as half-starved. There's a trail of silver paper behind me on the sidewalk, and malted milk balls are falling through my shaky fingers into the gutter. I do not bend to pick them up. I have fallen low, but not that low.

My mother has put me on something called the Josephine Lowman Nine-Day Diet, which she cut out of the *New York Post.* I am almost twelve years old, and I wear size 13, the largest girls' size there is. I am now taller than all the other girls in my school, and at the rate I am going, I will soon be the biggest teen-ager in the world. I will also have the biggest breasts—I'm already a B cup.

When I came out of the movie theater with my parents last Saturday night, pretending I was Ava Gardner, a man lurched toward me in the lobby, and my mother grabbed me by the wrist. "If I ever see you looking at a man like that . . ." My father looked at me sorrowfully. I'm still confused about this episode. I know I wasn't looking at anyone in particular, and I think it must have something to do with my breasts, which stick out in a presumptuous way despite anything I do to hide them. I've already heard loud wolf whistles on the post-office steps, whistles which filled me with delirious joy.

If I lose weight, I think, I will look more like a fashion model and less like the prostitute I undoubtedly will soon become.

My diet works like a charm. Each day's menu is printed in the newspaper. I eat only what's printed, and in nine days I lose five pounds. I feel grateful to Josephine Lowman, whoever she is. Then my mother suggests that I try for ten pounds, and I start the nine-day cycle all over again; she's saved the newspaper clippings. This time I am promised something extra as a reward—I forget what. A record? A baggy crew-neck sweater to cover the offending breasts?

Perhaps at this point I should mention that my mother, although slim, has a really large, enormous bust. She wears bras like girdles, with five hooks down the back. She puts little puffs of lamb's wool under the straps to ease the pressure on her shoulders. Whenever she takes a photo, she stands sideways holding her pocketbook in front of her, or else sits down behind a vase of flowers.

On my way to school at eight in the morning, I am already hungry. In the basement lunchroom, I open the meal that my mother has prepared. She's gotten up especially early to chop radishes and green peppers and mix them into a container of cottage cheese. She's wrapped it all up in a pretty flowered paper napkin— which unfortunately I can't eat—along with a plastic spoon. In the thermos is some bluish skim milk. I forget that I want to be a flat-chested size 9 and that I want my mother to love me. I think about taking the pennies out of my penny loafers and buying some chocolate mints.

Although I've sinned mostly in thought, at the end of the second nine days I've lost only two measly pounds. Still, my mother isn't discouraged. One more cycle, she promises, and we'll hit the ten-pound jackpot. Okay, I say, without making a fuss, I'll do it.

It's a problem with me that I never make a fuss. I always seem to be thinking about something else when my own fate is being discussed.

Before long I am getting up in the middle of the night and sneaking downstairs for some peanut butter to keep me going until breakfast. Heart pounding as I ease open the refrigerator door, I hastily lick the spoon and hide it in the back of a drawer.

A few days later I take the money I've been given to pay a library fine and squander it on two dripping slices of pizza. Worst of all, I abandon the library books, like some unwanted baby, on the floor of a telephone booth.

At about this time I begin investing my carfare in sweets. All the ensuing exercise doesn't help. By the twenty-seventh day, after diligent stuffing, I have gained back four pounds, for a net loss of three pounds. My mother is furious.

Scarlet-faced, I swear that I have never broken my diet—no, not even once.

During the next scene, my father, who is away much of the time, working in his plumbing-supply business, appears to learn about the diet for the first time.

"Diet? Who needs a diet? She's just perfect the way she is," he explains, seeking to soothe everyone's feelings. "Please, no more diets around here," he says. He wonders why my mother is so angry.

My mother puts me back on regular family rations. No more poached egg on protein bread, thank God. To be on the safe side, she also puts a combination lock on the kitchen cabinet holding bread, cereals, the pilot biscuits for her own modest snacks, and the peanut butter.

Without a diet, she says, she is afraid of what I will become.

Now something unusual and thrilling happens in my family; a Polish girl is coming to stay with us, a nineteen-year-old relative who needs a heart operation. She's the daughter of my mother's cousin—the only survivor of the European branch of the family. All the other Polish Jews—grandparents, aunts, uncles and cousins—were marched off to the railroad station by the Nazis with one suitcase apiece and never heard of again.

We make elaborate preparations for our visitor, whose name is Luba. My mother is busy for days beforehand, fixing up our guest room, cleaning and polishing. When Luba finally does appear on the dock, she is completely disappointing—as tiny as a mouse, pale and unresponsive. She's quickly whisked off to the hospital, where I'm too young to be welcome. After surgery, my mother devotedly visits Luba every day, carrying, in empty cottage cheese containers, little tidbits she has cooked.

When Luba returns to our house after her successful operation, she's no longer wan and washed out, but bright and vivacious. Although she looks delicate, with her little cherry mouth and translucent complexion, she's a powerhouse of nervous energy, greedily cramming a lifetime of pleasure into her few weeks in New York City.

Luba and my mother spend almost every afternoon together, while I am in school. They catch the show at the Radio City Music Hall and climb the Statue of Liberty. Because my mother thinks Luba's clothes look frumpy, they go off to Fulton Street to buy her a new outfit—a dainty silk organza dress with puffed sleeves and a sweetheart neckline. It's a size 5 and has a swooping, ruffled hemline. Luba also buys tiny ballet shoes with ankle straps, nylon stockings, and a narrow black velvet ribbon to wear around her neck. She enthusiastically tries on her new clothes in my room in front of my full-length mirror, while I stand nearby like a fence post.

Boxes and tissue paper litter my bed. My mother is excited; as she watches Luba twirl, her eyes gleam.

Later on my mother confesses to me that Luba has a little bit of "goyische taste." "After all, her father isn't Jewish. Still, it's a pleasure to shop with someone so easy to please. . . ."

One good thing—while they are gadding about, I get to see more of my father. I have to give him supper while Mother and Luba are out at a Broadway show. He seems pleased. Instead of reading the *Post* while eating, he asks me about my schoolwork. He doesn't usually ask, he says, because he has perfect confidence that I am doing well. In the same spirit, I ask him about plumbing supplies.

Luba and my mother go to Washington for two days. I will get my turn during Easter vacation, I am told, if I care for that sort of thing. "Actually, it was boring," my mother whispers reassuringly when they return. "I only ran here and there for Luba's sake."

I feel no anger toward my mother, but I develop a hatred for Luba. Her incomprehensible chatter, her sharp little nose, her high voice, her small, always-moving mouth, enrage me. We've tried a few exchanges which never lead anywhere, because Luba speaks little English, and I have no Polish. Her intense, mouse-eyed stare makes me uneasy.

"You go to the Freak Museum?" she asks.

"Freaks? Coney Island, you mean? No, not for a long time. You want to go to the boardwalk?"

"No, Freaks, Freak Museum." She jabs a skinny finger at my chest. "Artist."

Several years later, when I am in high school, I discover the existence of the Frick Collection.

A few days before Luba's departure, an unexpected check arrives from her mother, and she's out on a final orgy of buying: more nylons, Woolworth knickknacks for her friends, lipsticks and earrings. She's learned to take the bus to Bay Parkway and disappears for whole mornings by herself. One day she comes home with a fancy box of Barton's chocolates. For the first time, I hear words of adulterated praise from my mother.

"She could offer to share the candy," Mother says. "She's been eating our food night and day." The truth is, Luba eats far more than I do—whole quarts of chocolate ice cream, for instance—but she doesn't appear to have gained an ounce. Her trim waist sways fetchingly as she ascends the staircase with the candy.

For a moment, Mother and I are both annoyed at the thought of Luba upstairs, lolling on the fourposter bed which takes up most of the little guest room. With her feet up on the white snow-flake comforter, she is eating her way through truffles, chocolate cherries, coconut kisses, and caramel creams.

Another thing upsets my mother: Luba has not bought *her* any present. At the last minute, from her luggage, Luba produces a hideous purple china peacock to put on top of the piano.

Although the bird is the height of "goyische taste," my mother is appeased. She bakes a batch of Toll House cookies for Luba's final snack. Most of the cookies go into a tin for Luba to eat at her leisure on the boat. Mother gives me one while it is still warm, the chocolate bits still melting lusciously. Luba herself takes the remaining cookies upstairs to her room on a willow-ware plate, covered by a napkin. She places them carefully on the top of her bureau, then goes downstairs to watch television with my mother.

I am roaming around on the upper floor of our house just before going to bed. While my father snores in their room, I wander into Luba's room, homing in on the Toll House cookies.

After staring at the plate and lifting the napkin, I drift over to the closet to take a last look at Luba's pink organza dress—it will be packed first thing in the morning. When I glance at myself in Luba's oval mirror, the face about my white terrycloth bathrobe has a funny, pinched look.

Quickly I snatch one small, chipped cookie and rush back to my room to munch it, viciously. Then I return for a larger, perfect cookie and stand by the bureau, dreamily ingesting it. These cookies seem crispier than the one I was given. I select another large cookie. After successfully rearranging the whole pile for greater bulk, I eat it. Then I take another large one and eat it.

When I take a second look, I see that I may have gone too far. The pile looks shrunken. I may be able to get away with it, though. A person who can eat a whole box of Barton's chocolates by herself and consume whole quarts of ice cream is not going to have much feeling for the slight calibrations in a pile of cookies. I brush my teeth, get into bed, and turn out the light.

After several minutes of restless tossing, I realize that I am still close to starvation. If I am deprived of one more cookie, I shall go mad. I sneak back into Luba's room, grab a cookie at random and nibble it neatly around all the edges. When it is a normal-looking albeit much smaller cookie, I replace it. Then I tip-toe back to my room, close the door, and fall into a light, troubled sleep.

In the middle of the night, as I am dreaming dark, vengeful dreams, my door opens quietly. As my eyes fly open, I see Luba's slender figure in the light from the hallway. She is carrying a plate. I quickly shut my eyes and breathe deeply. She places the plate on my bedside table and tiptoes out.

As soon as I am alone, I reach out to examine the plate, although I already know what it is.

I am filled with deep humiliation and hatred.

So I have contaminated Luba's cookies! She no longer wishes to eat what I have defiled. I feel like jumping out of bed and flinging them back in her face.

In a few moments, however, the smell of the cookies begins to soothe me. A sort of anaesthesia takes hold of me. As I lie back on my pillow, holding the plate on my breast, I devour the whole pile, all of them, down to the last little grainy crumb. They are very delicious. I feel tranquil as I put down the plate and drop into a deep sleep.

When I awake at dawn, the plate is gone.

At the breakfast table, I examine Luba's face closely. She is her usual vivacious, insensitive self. She gives no hint of midnight happenings. It was all a dream, I pretend to myself thankfully.

After Luba left for Poland, my mother was a little depressed. Life seemed dull, so she took a trip to the mountains. When she turned the spotlight of her attention back on me I was no longer a child; I was a teenager. Elected editor of our class yearbook, I was busy choosing my staff and convening meetings. I dimly felt how lucky I had been, how peaceful it had been, to live for a time neglected in my own home.

We heard little of Luba after her return. She became a doctor and married well. According to my mother, she is unfailingly kind to her mother and has two handsome sons.

I now recognize Luba's act for one of kindness. She saw how deprived I felt and wanted me to have what I needed so desperately. Perhaps I will meet her someday to thank her, but in my proud, unregenerate heart I hope I never see her again—unless, of course, she has grown extremely stout in the meantime.

—Sondra Spatt Olsen

The Path of Excess

"The path of excess can lead to enlightenment."

—William Blake

The atmosphere is subdued in our household at the moment. I'm dieting again. No more time spent standing in front of the freezer scooping ice cream from the carton with a finger. No more glaze-outs over the stove tasting away the spaghetti sauce intended for the family dinner. It's half cups of raw vegetables, boiled eggs, vitamins, and a grim (possibly slim) future.

The children prefer life when I'm on one of my binges. I take them out for dessert and encourage them to order hot fudge, butterscotch or marshmallow sundaes. I don't tell them about the other flavors—after all, I eat their leftovers. I clip coupons from newspapers and take them to restaurants where families can gorge at two-for-the-price-of-one. I accept all lunch invitations and recently reached a zenith of some kind when I worked my way around a table finishing everyone's quiche. The children always like me, whatever shape I'm in. They hug me as I stand in front of the gas stove, burrowing their heads into the soft depths of my stomach. When we cuddle together on the settee, they fidget against me until their cheeks lie smooth against my breast, then sigh. My husband, from the depths of his introversion, reaches for me always.

I can't help believing there is a use for all this fat. Twenty years ago, *Life* magazine did a cover story on an unfortunate couple whose plane crashed, leaving them stranded in the frozen Alaskan wilderness. In the six weeks that passed before their rescue, their only sustenance was one rabbit which they caught and ate. Yet they survived. Although the couple credited their survival to God, doctors reported that neither of them would have endured had they not been overweight to start with.

I have a fantasy in which I am the sole passenger in an airplane, flown by a handsome pilot, forced to crash-land in the desert. As we stagger around the endless sands, I become slim and ethereal, while he becomes irritable and weak and finally faints away, muttering, "You've been excellent company. I can't understand how you can stay so even-tempered."

All the women's magazines at the supermarket checkout stands are full of luscious recipes, accompanied by the diet of the latest soon-to-be-very-rich doctor. The *National Enquirer* has a standing headline about diets. "At last, the eat all you want and get thin diet you've been waiting for, page 76." I look. It's eat all you want of raw Swiss chard. Now that's a wonderfully simple idea for a diet—prepare meals that are so repulsive they are impossible to eat. I can imagine next month's big story, "How the entire police force of Butte, Montana, lost 12,000 pounds on the Amazing Afghanistan Stuffed Goat's Bladder Diet."

My own instances of weight loss reveal a rapturous pattern. In my twenties I once fell in love so devastatingly I neither ate nor slept for three weeks. I would sit up all night breathing in the stars and smoking, until finally I became so thin that friends took me to a wise old doctor who pronounced me perfect, but in love. Another time I went without food for six days straight because a new acquaintance, challenging me with his charged eyes and holiness, said, "What, Jill, you couldn't manage to fast?" Recently I lost weight when the handsome contractor who won the bid to build a room onto our house fell in love with me. I preened in my velvet house gown and grew thin playing the ideal mother and witty wife while he lurked outside windows waiting for glimpses of me. My husband obliviously accepted the unrequested closet, heater and French window he built in for us.

In contrast, I put on weight when unhappy or bored. Once I put fifteen pounds on my small frame in three weeks when my car was broken down and I was trapped in the house with my three small children.

I put on weight when living in Greece. The social appreciation of plumpness made it so easy. Once a man confessed in halting English, "I don't mind skinny girls like you." I felt wonderful as I reached for more baklava. The women there encouraged me to eat by saying, "You're married, aren't you? Then why worry about how much you eat?" Those Old World women were guerrilla eaters on the domestic front!

I put on weight the last time my father stayed with me. My father, a widower of eighty, is vivacious company. His humor is old-fashioned sexist, and though I tried not to be affected by it, eventually I felt undermined and started sneaking away from him to the kitchen for treats, just as my mother had done.

Nearly all my mother's vigor, high intelligence and capability went into organizing meals. When I was young we spent our summers at the seaside in England. My mother and her sisters, who were big, stalwart women, would wait until the seasonal visitors had returned to their hotels for lunch, then disappear behind the changing curtains in the back of our beach bungalow. After a lot of guffaws and exclamations, my aunts and my mother would reappear in large bathing suits with "skirts." They would trip awkwardly across the sands while my father would shout, "There go the heavies for Cherbourg." (At the continental landing in World War II the lighter craft landed at Normandy, whereas the heavier ships, which drew more water, had to use the harbor at Cherbourg.) My mother and her sisters would giggle nervously and collapse into the sea like grateful seals.

I have an image of myself as an octopus. I am standing on two of my legs while all the other legs are throwing food at my stomach—odd peanut butter and jelly scraps, half cartons of yogurt—backing me against a rock wall. I have tried to imagine this octopus *thin*, venturing out into the swim. Great sharks and barracudas sweep down the corridors of Ocean, engulfing her in their wake. When these great fish finally notice her, they scoop her up and take her to their caves, where they praise and frighten her.

In my fantasy, the Thin Octopus asks the Fat Octopus, "Why is it the Great Streamlined Fish of Ocean don't do that to you when you make your brief sorties out into the swim of things?"

My Fat Octopus replies, "These powerful fish make room for me nonchalantly, uninterestedly. My fat announces that I am out of the sexual swim and makes me almost invisible, though sometimes I feel faint from lack of acknowledgment."

"But in ecstatic states you lose your fat as fast as can be!" says the Thin Octopus. "Couldn't you make yourself strong, to cope with stress, rather than so fat that you are unable to make the moves that bring about changes?"

"I would like to, but I don't want to be like you, Thin Octopus. You are too weak to say 'no' to any passing barracuda."

I don't have to be a puny octopus at all. I could be a

super fish, muscular and healthy, anxious to get out in the swim, streaming down the corridors of Ocean, flipping her tail at the other fish, giving them the fish eye, nudging them painfully in the fin if she wants them out of her way, sending out "Don't come into my lane" signals even when the shark is way off. My sleek fish could become a positive bully, and though my absolute standards of fair play think this is a dreadful way to behave, I like to think of her at the crossroads of the great swim, challenging all comers.

—Jill Jeffery

The Diet

"For instance," she said as she sat across from me consuming a big Coca-Cola glass full of melting ice cream, "for breakfast yesterday morning I had two eggs, boiled. Then, not being quite satisfied with that, I had two more eggs, boiled. I guess I should have realized right then about what kind of day it would be—the pattern. Then I had a small peanut butter san, minus the bread, and later a small little bit of Quaker Granola cereal I stole from one of my housemates' cupboards. I had that with a quarter cup of nonfat milk, and with this sort of extended breakfast I had two cups of coffee, black. This breakfast seemed to do it, but I *did* have some snacks throughout the day. Six cups of coffee altogether, black. And a small little bit of milk that I drank, taken from a roommate's carton in the fridge, just a swallow or two, and . . . ah . . .

let me see, oh, and one teaspoon of honey. This got me through the day—until six o'clock.

"Then I think the problem was that, you know, it gets to be dinnertime, and everybody else is eating and you're not, like it's a very deeply ingrained habit to *eat* at dinnertime—it has all sorts of psychological flotsam and jetsam attached to it, love and family and security, the hearth and all that. The problem is, when you're not going to eat dinner, what do you do with that time? The time when everybody else is *eating?* Well, at about six I met Marge and she said, 'You've got to eat *something,* even if it's just a sandwich.' So we went to a Hofbrau on Clement. She ordered a pitcher of beer and a big beautiful pastrami, so I ordered a pastrami san too, and drank a quart and a half of beer with it.

"For some reason this sandwich triggered off something in me. I don't know why it is, but this has happened to me before; that's why when I go on a diet it's best for me to just drink liquids; then this *craving* for all sorts of yummy foods doesn't get me. Well, I gave in just a little and ordered a half pint of potato salad. Then as we walked back to the apartment we passed a Baskin-Robbins. I had to have one. I had a chocolate chip and praline, double header, on a sugar cone. When I got home I ate a small little box of Cheezits that belonged to another of my housemates, and then I had two glasses of milk. I couldn't stop, I was so hungry, so I went out and brought back a pint of chocolate almond ice cream and ate it all. When I got back from the store, after the pint, I had a peanut butter san, this time with the bread, and one spoonful of malted milk powder on top—it wasn't mine—the malted milk—someone else in the house had it in their food cabinet and I just snuck a little of it.

"By this time it was eleven-thirty at night and I was feeling very, very sleepy from the last five hours of eating. I felt guilty when I polished off Mike's—that's another of my roommates—anchovy and pepperoni pizza which he had half of left over in the fridge. I was depressed. I tried to reorient myself. I went in and fixed myself up a platter of healthy things, vegetables and stuff. Some carrot sticks, celery stalks, radishes, sweet gherkins, pickled hot-mix vegetables, spiced cauliflower, cucumber slices, that sort of thing, all on a platter, and I ate it while I watched the Billy the Kid ballet on Channel 9. As I say, I was depressed, although not as disgusted with myself as I thought I should feel—I'd only been on the diet for a couple of days.

"But that food, you know, it makes you sleepy; it acts like a soporific and you can sleep, go right off to sleep after a binge, although it's hard to wake up in the morning. That's when you feel kind of sick; you feel like you're a revolting tub, like you have carboholic poisoning or something. But the worst thing is the feeling that you really don't have any control over yourself at all. It's a feeling of impotence about whether or not *you, conscious you*, really have anything to say about who is running your physical self. It's almost like some other personality has taken control over you, and that personality wants to see you weigh a ton for all it's concerned. It doesn't *like* you—it wants to make you ugly, and it can never be satisfied.

"But I read once, you know, in a book called *The Fifty Minute Hour*, about this horrendously fat woman who ate immense amounts of food on binges. Then finally she locked herself in her apartment for a week. Her apartment was filled to the top with all kinds of food, canned, fresh and frozen—she must have prepared for this one good—and she ate day and night. Hundreds of bananas, pears, apples, cakes, cookies, ice cream, cartons of cream and chocolate drinks, candies of every kind, fudge by the boxes—she even ate a couple of cartons of Ayds candies that she had left over from a diet that her psychiatrist had put her on. She had mountains of canned stuff that she would just open with the can opener and stuff in her face uncooked because she ate so much so fast during the first days of her orgy. After a while she couldn't get up off the couch anymore and she just threw the peelings, empty cans, boxes, cartons, wrappings and whatever over her shoulder all over the floor of the place. She had planned it so when she couldn't get up any longer, something edible was close enough to crawl to.

"Well, the psychiatrist went to her apartment when she didn't show for her weekly appointment. He had to break the door down to get in—she was in a coma—and the shrink could barely stand the smell of the place, or even hardly get through all the food remains to get to her immense body—she was well over three hundred fifty pounds. Her apartment was one gigantic refuse heap—like some organic instant archeological midden hidden away in this apartment complex of modern-day America.

"Well, when her shrink finally got to her through it all, and found a phone to call the ambulance, he saw that *her eyes were gone.* He *couldn't see her eyes at all;* they had completely disappeared into the fat of her face. She was horribly bloated, like somebody who has been floating dead in the river a long time. She had passed out with a half-eaten banana in one hand and a piece of Boston cream pie in the other.

"She lived, though—and the psychiatrist finally cured her after about a year of intense therapy. *He* said she did it because subconsciously she wanted to get pregnant and this was her way of simulating pregnancy. She'd never even had a sexual relationship, of *any* kind, in her entire life. I wish he had let her tell why *she* thought she did it; it would have been interesting to see what she said about it. I mean, I know with me, I've never wanted to get pregnant, *consciously or subconsciously*, you know?" she said, finally polishing off the glass of melted Neapolitan, lifting it almost vertical, and letting the last swallow slide sensuously down the side of the glass into her open mouth.

—*Penny Skillman*

Eating as Metaphor, Part 1: HUNGER

"Going to sleep alone is lonely. But going to sleep with someone who tears your heart out is worse."

—*My mother*

Hunger

Most of us walk around hungry; some of us will die hungry. Subtle in its manifestations, nonphysical hunger can take the form of a vague disturbance, an amorphous dissatisfaction, a feeling that there has to be more to life than what we've known or had. If we interpret the hunger literally, we can use food or drink to satisfy it, or, more to the point, to dull it. Nonphysical hunger is difficult to tolerate because it is uncomfortable to feel. If our attempts at avoiding it are unsuccessful, the inner gnawing grows, and the discomfort gets more and more unbearable.

Some people feel deprived because they are withering at their jobs; they are hungry for work that uses their talents. Some people are living the way they've been told they should, and have never stopped to question whether or not they are happy or fulfilled. When something happens to interrupt their lives—a tragedy, an accident—they begin to question the importance of how they fill their time. Some hungers may reach deeper: they may indicate a need for a transcendental or a spiritual pursuit of some sort. Many people are troubled by a need to be assertive, to say no when they feel no, to take care of their own wants instead of seeming always to have to look out for others.

At a given moment, our hunger might indicate a yearning as simple as asking to be held—or as complex as the necessity to examine a set of attitudes and responses we have developed in the past that are no longer effective in our present situation. Some key issues may be: the manner in which we express our vulnerability and ask for help; our ability to set limits of behavior and accept the limits of others; the appropriateness of the people with whom we have become intimately involved—their capability and willingness to respond to and support us emotionally, sexually, intellectually; our mistrust of men or women because of a hurtful situation in the past.

Hunger is deeply personal—it is the unanswered side of our dreams; it is born of the need for completion, fulfillment and serenity.

When we become aware of what we are hungry for, we can begin to seek the appropriate nourishment.

Many compulsive eaters believe that their hunger would be relieved if they were thin. They think that being thin would make everything all right; that being thin would make them happy. I've worked with many people who refuse to believe that their pain would not disappear if they were thin. Despite the fact that most of them have already been thin once or twice, the tenacity with which they hold onto "thinness as happiness" prevents them from getting to the root of their hunger.

It is not surprising that thinness and happiness have become synonymous. With models and TV and movie stars being thin, with insurance charts scaled down to minimal measurements, with elegant clothes coming only in small sizes, our society's ideal figure has become a bony one. And because most of us are hungry and are searching for a way to appease our hunger, we are open targets for solutions presented to us in glossy packages.

When you believe your hunger is related to something as controllable as the shape of your body, you don't have to undergo the sometimes lengthy and often painful questioning of other things about yourself. You don't have to come face to face with empty dreams or the lack of fulfillment you experience in your work and/or relationships. You can decide that your troubles are weight-related—and then you can continue to eat compulsively. Never attaining permanent status as a thin person, you continue to strive for a goal that you will never reach because you keep standing in your own way. Reaching the goal would mean facing the unsettling conclusion that being thin had little to do with being happy, and that all the striving that went into the attainment of this goal did not bring you any closer to a sense of inner peace.

Rather than experience this disillusionment, many people gain back the weight they've spent years taking off. And so the merry-go-round continues—a different diet, another doctor, a new organization.

If you have invested a lot of time and money in efforts to get thin, it can be devastating to find that you are still plagued by a hunger you cannot define. Yet this is a hunger, Thomas Merton says, "that will never be satisfied with any created thing."

Although it is understandable that you try to satisfy it with being thin, it is imperative that you see the futility of your attempts so that you can break free from the cycle of compulsive eating.

This doesn't mean losing twenty pounds and *then* thinking about your "indefinable hunger." That's just a trick you play to perpetuate your belief that you cannot be happy *until* you are thin.

Given the values of the society we live in, with the emphasis on gloss and external appearances, the concept of a hunger that cannot "be satisfied with any created thing" is not easy to incorporate. For this, you must rely on your own experiences: Being thin is a "thing." Has any "thing" you've ever obtained brought you truly long-lasting satisfaction? Is it not true that the excitement of a "thing" is in the desiring of it, and that once it is yours, your focus changes to the next "thing" you don't have? Because being thin is not easily recognizable as a thing—the way a house, a dress, or a car is—it may be difficult to see the validity of this reasoning. And yet, if you think about it, being thin is not an inner state of being: it is something your *body* isn't. It is external; its value is created by the society and the times.

It is not my intent to negate the value of created things. We depend on them for survival; they make life easier and aesthetically more pleasing. It *is* my intent, however, to clarify the distinction between hungers that can be satisfied by created things and hungers that can't.

If being thin is, for you, the goal on which you pin your well-being, then you are probably hungry for something less tangible. You are probably depriving yourself in other areas of your life.

Are you willing to risk forsaking your belief that being thin is equated with happiness in order to discover the root of your hunger?

Are you willing to discover how you keep yourself deprived?

Days Alone Come Down to This

Days alone come down to this. I work, I write, and the sun goes down. Then, if I don't have a group in the evening, I don't always know what to do with myself. Maybe I'll call Nancy upstairs, call her and have her down for an hour or two. I see myself sitting in the rocking chair, Nancy on the bed. I see myself listening to her and thinking about my writing. No, I won't call Nancy. Go to a movie, then. Katharine Hepburn is playing in *Mary, Queen of Scots*. I love Hepburn; it would be a pleasure to see her, but a distraction. From what? From following myself into the center, which I keep trying to avoid. I don't know what to do when

I get done. So I distract myself by calling a friend, seeing a movie.

I remember now why I ate.

Last Thursday morning I had returned from Tom's house facing the possibility of our relationship's ending. The ache in my chest had spread to my shoulders, neck, stomach. I was also hungry, so I prepared my usual breakfast. As I sat at the kitchen table, I thought, "I don't want to have to get up from this table and go on to the next thing. I hurt too much." I looked down at my plate; only one dried pear left. But lots more in the refrigerator, a whole bag full. "I could eat all day. That way I wouldn't have to think about anything else. Tom's face; the way the light hits his beard in the morning, streaming through the red and white hairs."

"Snap out of it," I told myself. "Stop dwelling on his face." I can't.

What about the pears? It would be so easy to let the morning fade noiselessly into afternoon while I sat here chewing and chewing. It would give me something to do. I could eat till I couldn't eat; then I could sleep. When I awoke the pain in my stomach would be louder than the one in my chest. I could drown the ache, wash it over with waves and waves of nausea, transfer my despair to the physical level. Food magic. Until the hollowness sucked me cold like a vacuum and I needed relief again.

Days alone come down to this: Propelling myself through a labyrinth of walls whose texture changes, paths whose scenery varies, I follow the tangled forest of my mind. And then I get to the center and then I run. I talk I leave I eat but I run. The center—steel gray, I imagine, with lacy edges—but the center of what? Of whatever I eat to avoid. The center, a reservoir of my life's experiences, a storehouse of images, tears, knowledge, wisdom. The center, the ineffable center of me. Where is it? In my chest? My stomach? My brain?

Wherever it is, it is waiting; it is hungry. Like a baby bird whose mouth waits to be filled, it is hungry. The hunger stretches across miles, closes in on itself and begins again. Like a circle with a million circles inside of it, my hunger, stark and raw, waits for me at the center.

When I am standing at the rim, it looks like darkness, like the gulf between two bodies or two thoughts, between two breaths. There is always the chance that the next word may not arise, that the bodies may not come together, or that the next breath will not be taken. Terrified of taking that chance, I talk I leave I eat but I run. I am terrified of leaping so far—what if my legs won't hold me? What if I make the leap and all that's there is silence, separation and death?

It's safer, yes, it's safer to stay hungry. Like a fist in my stomach, my hunger opens and closes. Sometimes I can ignore it. *And* there is always food. One dried pear after another, chewing and chewing and chewing, sitting at the kitchen table until the sun goes down and the shadows lengthen and there is nothing else to do but go to bed. In the morning I am an echo of myself.

The others—what do they do with their hungers? The voice at the center of the vortex that calls them, beckons them to follow its spiraling down, down to the starkness, the rawness? They may drink or take drugs, or they eat; oh yes, they eat. It's all the same. We all run. We are all afraid of our own hungers.

Except the ones who aren't. The madmen, the artists, the saints. They walk right into the starkness. They absorb their grief. They become, they actually become, the space between one breath and another. The madmen stay mad because they are caught in the eye of the center, whirling. They become so enmeshed in the heart of the darkness that they think that's all there is. They leap *into*, but do not know to leap out of. The artists, the saints get to the other side. No longer afraid of their own hungers, they seem to live at the center of a sparkle that brightens and dims according to a natural rhythm. But even the madmen are ahead of us: at least they leap. We would rather remain hungry and afraid. We would rather turn to food or drugs or drink that dulls the call, never reaching the loamy hungers inside.

The drive to eat compulsively is not about food. It is about hungers. The hungers of regret and sorrow, of unspoken anger, unrealized dreams; the hungers of your own potential that are waiting to be filled, like a baby bird's mouth. The more you run from them, the more they threaten to overtake you, consume you, so the more you run from them. Something in you—the voice of your hungers—does not want you to die without having realized your own uniqueness, so it calls to you. When you don't listen, it screams at you. When you run, it follows you. Trying to escape from it is like trying to escape from your own shadow.

The more you run, the more frightened you become. Because then you have to deal with the problem you've created along the way: the ten or twenty or thirty pounds you've gained. Problems that arise from running are only symptoms of the underlying hungers. But they become realities in themselves that must be dealt with—so the focus gets transferred from the psychic to the physical level.

Yet when you stop running, you stop being afraid. It turns out that the fear of hunger is worse than the hunger itself. Because the hunger, when you're in it, is just hunger. Not frightening, not anything but hunger. Out of the experience of it, a way to fill it becomes apparent. When you are being afraid of it, you can't focus on ways to ease it. Fear is all you know— wild fear that sends you running, trembling in ten different directions, all of which are an attempt to avoid, not to fulfill, the hunger.

When you stop running, you become part artist, part madwoman, part saint.

Days alone come down to this. A choice between running and standing still. Yesterday I wrote until the sun went down. And then I didn't know what to do. I was slammed up against myself and I wanted to escape, climb the walls of the labyrinth. Wedged into an empty space, I felt myself slipping into the steel-gray center, and I wanted to flail my arms and legs, get back outside again. But since I was writing about hungers, I decided to follow the beat of the silence. In my rocking chair, I watched. The wind chimes brushed together softly; a mocking-bird sang out. I waited, and watched myself waiting. I wanted to run, to eat, to call someone—even the operator at my answering service would do. Break the stillness, the deafening aloneness, the movement into the center of hunger. As I rocked back and forth, back and forth, and the chair creaked against the floor, the sound of my own sighs startled me. A spider weaved its way over my desk. I let myself down into the space between thoughts. The steel-gray center became fluid and weightless, and then I wasn't waiting anymore, wasn't fright-ened anymore. There was no trying, no struggle. It seemed as though the shape of the hungry space receded where I stuck out and stuck out where I receded, so that when I slipped into it, we fit. And like puzzle pieces that, when assembled, create an image, a visual unity that makes you forget about the individual parts, when I slipped into the hungry space, it and I—we—became a third thing, a felt unity. Me became me being me. Not me being afraid or me being hungry but me being what makes me me. In the crevices between unscheduled moments—the moments I am most fearful of—the background noise is dimmed to such a low level that I can unfold myself if I dare. I become authentic. Am I most fearful, then, of becoming uniquely myself? Of the power that would ensue if I weren't constantly trying to talk myself out of being myself? Are the empty spaces empty because I refuse to join my edges with their recessions? Probably.

Yesterday, as I sat in the rocking chair, in the silence, the image of a bird came in. A Japanese paper bird, delicately folded in origami style. The beak was well defined, the head small and unobtrusive; the wingspan was glorious, streaked with blues and purple. A long and graceful body edged out into a tail with three distinct feathers. I thought to unfold it. Then the voice of fear: "No. If you do that, you'll never put it back together. Keep it in one piece." Rocking back and forth, I argued with myself: "Unfold it, see how it works." "Leave it alone." "Go ahead." "If you unfold the bird, you will be left with empty spaces; then what will you do?" I looked again at the bird, decided to unfold it. First the beak, then the head. After that, the body, unfolding back in on itself more and more until I got to the wings.

And when I unfolded them, first one and then the other, I saw that the space between the wings, like the space between breaths, contained the secret of how to fly.

I Don't Eat Potatoes

I'm counting out peanuts for Mac. He can't do it himself— this you must understand—and yet they must be counted; so I count. It doesn't take long, but today I'm distracted, must begin again. Maybe it's this corner of the kitchen: the phone's right here, and I keep thinking it's about to ring. *Hello—twelve, thirteen—oh, hi—fourteen* (I'd finish the last half dozen in my head). *Fourteen what?* they'd ask. *Peanuts,* I'd say. *I'm counting them out for Mac.* They'd pretend not to hear right, say *What?* think I'm kidding, make me feel caught in the act of someone's insanity. But that's nonsense, and I resent it; they proba- bly do worse for theirs—like roll each of his socks up with its mate so he won't have to hunt in a deep, dark drawer. If they give me a hard time about this peanut business, I can always remind them of the many acts we all religiously perform in full faith and absence of mind—like asking if he's got the tickets in his pocket, serving saccharin along with his strudel.

You see, Mac's afraid of dying. It's the truth. He came home last Thursday and started this guessing game the way he loves to because I always get impatient and make a mess of them. (Mac says I've got a sense of humor, all right; I just don't know where to draw the line.) The game: Well, *he* says, "I went to see Michael today for a complete physical." I nod my head in approval. "And what do you think Michael said to me, Sylvia?" he asks.

"I don't know," I say. "I give up."

"Just guess," he says.

So I guess. I guess: "Michael said he's never seen a sounder specimen in his life!" Mac shakes his head. "Michael said your heart's as strong as espresso." Mac shakes his head. "Michael said it wouldn't kill you to lose a couple of pounds around the middle."

"Michael *said*," Mac says, "if I don't stop eating and drinking and lose some weight I'll die."

"Well, we all gotta go sometime." That's what I said. I don't know why—it was stupid—but it's just that I know Michael and the way he exaggerates. And knowing Mac and the way he loses perspective, I thought: Make a little joke and maybe he'll chuckle and stop worrying about the fact that he's not going to live forever.

Mac didn't chuckle. He just said, "And Michael said I should tell *you* that you're doing me no favor matching me drink for drink and cooking those magnificent briskets and—"

So I was thinking: Of course—how could I have been so blind? Why didn't I think of it?—It's all *my* fault he's not going to live forever. But Mac looked truly worried, so

I went to him with arms wide to hug him and tell him I loved him even though I never did know where to draw the line; but he gave me his back and was out the door.

So I decided to cook the chicken that night instead of saving it for the next night's company. I roasted it with carrots and onions and potatoes, and stewed some prunes and apricots. I took out the Brie so it wouldn't be cold. I'd serve Brie for dessert, with apples: Mac loves to feel continental.

"Sylvia," he shouts, halfway in the door, *"what smells!* Are you trying to kill me?" He often says that. It means, You're better than Julia Child. But *this* time he meant no flattery.

"I'm trying to love you," I said, "but you're making it difficult."

"You're trying to kill me! Fat, Fat—I'm a fat, unhealthy man."

"Mac, you still gotta eat. It's chicken, not lamb or lasagna. It's fruit and cheese for dessert."

"Sylvia, did you ever hear of cholesterol?"

Well, Mac ate his share, all the time muttering how I was trying to kill him—as if he really believed it. So I'm counting peanuts, to show him—as if after seventeen years he should still need proof—to show him I don't want him to die.

The truth is, I don't mind this counting. Six weeks? Ten? I can hardly remember, but I haven't missed a day, and have refrained from parceling them out in advance. Each day I count, and it reminds me how well we understand each other. If he simply said he was going to try to cut down on his peanut intake—how could he know for sure, how *empty* the jar was when he started, how *full* when he locked it back in the liquor closet and pocketed the key? If he made a pact to allow himself a single handful—well, I know Mac—he'd take up piano again, just to stretch his reach. And twenty, though it sounds like a lot, when it comes to peanuts, is, as they say, peanuts. He—we together—used to eat half a jar.

But the question remains: Why can't he count out his own? And the answer is—it's so obvious it's hard to explain. I mean, I feel instinctively that it makes sense, that he couldn't do it himself. It would seem as strange as my thinking of a number and then trying to guess it; or blindfolding myself and spinning myself before setting myself out to pin the tail on the donkey. *I* must do it for the same reason he must massage my charley horse even when it's in a place I can reach. In marriage we vow to support each other's *mishegas*. And besides, this counting is interesting in ways I hadn't imagined. At first I thought that in a few days I'd be able to make a fist and reach in and come out with twenty little elephant's delights every time; but then I remembered Darwin and realized that peanuts, being natural, are subject to variation and mutation; and *then* I thought that because of probability, maybe the deformities in any one handful would balance out those in any other; in the end, I decided to count every time.

Still, sometimes when I'm counting I start to miss those days with him in the brown chair and me in the green one and between us the end table supporting a lamp, two drinks, and a jar of peanuts. And because of probability and general gluttony, we'd often reach in together and knock knuckles and play fingzies and sometimes—at least once—I remember he clawed me and brought my hand to his mouth. "My, what salty thumbs you have," he growled. "The better to keep you hooked," I growled back. And I remember that, at least once, sharing the peanuts drove us to bed without our dinner. Kim wasn't home. She must have been at camp. It was hot. He undressed me in the hallway. I'd gladly let him do it again: my blouse downstairs, my brassiere on the landing, my pants at the top of the stairs. So what if I'm no Twiggy? It's just that Mac has changed since he's gotten so thin. Oh, he's no Twiggy either, but he's on his way—and he's less aggressive. Maybe because he eats so little meat. Maybe because he's tired from his sit-ups and push-ups and chin-ups on the bar across the door. No wonder he doesn't have any *oomph* left for me. It's grotesque the way he loves his life. I once read that in a book. The line isn't original, but the idea—the linkage of the line with that man in the living room, taking off his shoes, waiting for his Tanqueray, bone dry, up, with an olive, and his twenty dry-roasted peanuts—that's original. Well, let him wait. I can't find the gin. Let him meditate. Did it ever occur to him I might be dying too? It never occurred to me, but I'm not much thinner than he used to be, and I think it's only fair he should have asked.

They're out running—Mac and Kim, and I don't mean jogging, but running. The world is running, and running fast. I see them when I'm driving—everyone: the fat, thin, frog princes, fillies, studs, shepherds, mutts, rabbis, legislators—holding their chins high, their eyes skimming just above my hood with that pained ecstatic look which makes me weak and hungry. I step on the gas. I can't wait to get home for something to eat. Mac used to have to remind me it was time for peanuts and martinis. Now that he's no longer addicted—does it only when in the mood and nobody need count—now it's up to me to remind myself. I've adjusted; I never forget, though I miss those fights about who ate the last one or who ate more or whether this drink was number two or three. Now I could drink a dozen and not get a rise out of tight-lipped Mr. Trim. *Live and let live:* the motto of the younger generation; and the thinner Mr. Ponce de Leonovitz gets, the more he thinks he's one of them.

When Kim suggested I run with them, I pointed with my eyes to my *zaftig* self, and she said, "Well, you gotta start somewhere." I might have considered it, if only to make it a family affair; but Mac, who in the old days—don't ask me when—would have said, *Come on, you old bag of bulge. The world is waiting for you, YOU, to run, and we won't take no for an answer*—this new Mac said, "Kim, don't hassle your mother. When she's ready to run, she'll run. Let's go; I'm in a rush."

That's Mac these days: busy, busy, dates at the club, hardly has time to sit down and eat his dinner. Or maybe it's just that I use the wrong kind of flour, or oil, or proportion of *yin* to *yang*. If only he'd lend me those health and longevity books, instead of hiding them under the mattress as if they were *Fanny Hill*. He likes his side of the mattress, clings to it as if he can't bear to be near my thick side, reminder of his lost flesh.

I'm cooking a dinner I think they'll like: sea bass stuffed like James Beard suggests, with onions, celery, green pepper, bread crumbs, thyme, and almonds. Brown rice, salad, and *challah*. It's Friday.

They're banging up the porch steps, laughing—laughing as if they've been racing. "Hi, Mom. We're home." They smell of sweat and turning apples and the wet dirt and dry leaves they drag in with their fancy sneaker soles. They're racing up the stairs, laughing, fighting to claim the first shower. I put the bread in the oven. It won't be long before they come down, clean and glowing. I'll let Kim light the candles, recite the prayer. I'm not in the mood. She's fifteen, already a woman. My breath smells of Brie. I'm not in the mood.

He's counting. Ask him, he'll deny it. He'll say, *Why, I'm not even looking her way.* But I tell you he knows how many by this shadow that fans the carpet. It's the mark of my hand that has described the arc from dish to

mouth, twenty-eight times, now twenty-nine. The others
don't count—it's not polite; though me, I watch them, and
don't understand: They're not eating. There are peanut,
chip, canapé dishes on every table—untouched. They
discuss, laugh, nod their heads; they're engaged. But as
for Mac? Listen: they're calling his name. That's how I
know he's counting. There it is again: "Mac"—as if he
had to be snapped out of some preoccupation. *Shame
on you, Mac; those are your friends. Answer them. What
do you think of the price of soybeans?* See now, he's
blinked. He's back, right there, turning red, silently god-
damning me for distracting him from the conversation.
Well, it's not my fault he never was very good at doing
two things at once. Even in bed, it was a stroke here, rub
there, one place at a time. That was funny. It made me
love him. But maybe he's blushing for *me,* embarrassed
by *my* not mingling, not nodding, not laughing, just eating and drinking. Well, why doesn't he stand up, in front
of everyone—why doesn't he stamp his foot and say
he's had enough? If only he'd grab the dish and fling it
through the window. It would be major. Our friends
wouldn't understand; we wouldn't be invited to any more
of these parties. If only he'd pull one out of my mouth. I'd
bite him, make him bleed; I'd scream and cry. I know
that would help. If only he'd give me the evil eye—the
one I gave him when he scratched his wasp sting. He's
gotta do something, anything but this nothing, this not
counting, not seeing my shadow, my eating, me—oh, did
you think for a second he was distracted from the conversation because of my eating? No—it's just that he's
working on his serve, or jumping rope in his head.

It's me who's counting; trying not to, but it's like trying
not to think of an elephant. I say to myself: Now your
hand's in the dish, feel the metal, how cold, and the
peanuts—they're fewer. Your hand is in the dish. This

has happened before. How many times? You don't know. But I do. I know. Thirty-two, thirty-three. There's no turning back. If only he'd remember how I counted for him: hefty Mac with his hairy rolls and flabby jowls, fat Mac who couldn't touch his toes; how I stood by the window in the late afternoon sun and counted because he was weak and loved his peanuts.

Let's go. I must give him the signal it's time to leave. He'll know what I mean. We understand each other; we've been doing this for years. And he's probably as anxious to go as I am. He probably has a date at the club. I hope Kim has a date too. (If they're out late I'll drive to "John's" for ice cream.) I want no one home. I'm hungry. I've had too much to drink. If someone is there I won't get enough.

He's sleeping. He sleeps like a rock. The thinner he becomes and the more he runs, the harder the rock of his sleep. He never wakes—a blessing. If he opened his eyes and saw mine he might remember. That happens: in the middle of the night people wake; they don't know where they are, but they remember where they've been. Then he might reach out, graze through folds of bedding hunting for my shoulder. He might "X" his calf over mine, or press the cold gold band on his fourth knuckle into my hip. Or grumble about a dream: red cliffs, cows flying; or a nightmare: the commies—they're stealing his ice crea ... But there's no need to worry. I could be right here with another man and he wouldn't stir. Look: his eyelids don't flutter; he's not even dreaming. And I'm alone, not here with another man, but with me—as big as two—still, double that I am, I can't manage to keep myself company. Why can't he think of some reason to change this night-time arrangement: his back, his skin, some allergy? Why must he insist on ignoring what's happening? He should spend the night out, or bring her home to dinner, or leave. Instead, I leave. That is, I leave the bed. It happens like this: After he topples like a boulder into sleep, I drift off into my childhood Isadora Duncan dreams. I am she and just as slim in a gossamer gown, peeking out from between two large cypresses, my feet in a damp mossy forest—she's like me, with red hair and green eyes, and I'm *Sylvia:* "woman from the forest." Or, I'm a tall, thin little girl dancing in front of my parents' company. All day I polished the silver with Mommy. Pink polish that came in a jar and turned gray on the silver. She let me taste everything she was cooking. She let me lick the batter off the beaters. Now I'm in my nightie. I've bounced down the stairs with clean teeth, ready to give kisses good-night. Daddy sits down at the piano and plays a Russian tune. First it's slow, calling for a princess in a tutu. But I'm no ballerina, so Daddy speeds up, and now I can dance like I am—large and wild, stamping and spinning until I fall on the rug, dizzy, and giggling; and every mommy and daddy kisses pretty little tall skinny Sylvia a sweet dream kiss. And then Daddy carries her upstairs to bed.

When I awake—because those pretty dreams are disturbing and not as nice as they sound—I masturbate. Right here at his side. He never wakes. If he did it wouldn't matter, because he wouldn't let on. Often he snores. I rub to the in and out of his snoring, to the rhythm of the man who'll never enter me again. I can't imagine it. This hard tight muscle of a man inside this woman with flesh sprawling in every direction. How does he imagine it? Not at all. What if this belly were his child? Sometimes I forget, look down, say "Hi, there." She kicks. He used to say he wanted me fiercely then. But now he won't stay awake long enough to give any such thought a stretch of brain to clamp into. At least I try to imagine. It's important to try, not to lose hold.

I'm sick and want to throw up. But what if he heard retching and got up and found his wife vomiting into the toilet—her red hair soiled, her fat forehead sweaty, her knees trembling? Surely he'd love me—or pity me or something. But he won't wake, hear, find, feel. If he heard, he'd turn over. He needs his sleep; and as for fat people, they deserve what they get—sinful abusers of God's beauty.

Now Mac is like a rock beside me and I will get out of bed. I'll put on my green silk kimono, the one with the embroidered birds that fits and makes good fashion sense with this greasy limp hair and fish-white skin. It becomes the witch who thumps down all eighteen steps and sits at the bottom to catch her breath. Where is it? She can't remember. The broom closet? She goes to check. No, not there. The ice-skate bin? She checks, but no. Under the sink? No. The laundry room? Yes, of course, somewhere down in the basement. The witch thumps down to the laundry room and checks behind the washer and yes, and in the storage room, yes, and in the camp trunk, under the shorts and polo shirts taped with her daughter's name. In the garment bags, the nonperishables, the items that won't absorb the smell of mothballs: the vacuum-packed nuts, the biscuits from England, sardines from Norway, the raspberry jam, the candied ginger, the figs. But here behind the washer is chutney. That doesn't make sense: chutney belongs in the storage room. Maybe she heard someone coming and had to rush. There's avocados in the storage—that's a mistake too—and peanut brittle in the laundry, and in the trunk—she wanted to put in the things she loves best: the animal crackers, the braided licorice, the salami, the caramels—but here there are Grape-Nuts, and they're not her favorites—they belong in the storage room, or behind the washer; she must have heard footsteps and been in a rush, and now where will she eat? The laundry room first, or the trunk, or one item from each in a triangle so her legs won't fall asleep? She'll have to make sure to finish in time to climb the two flights and get into bed and shut her eyes before Mac's alarm rings.

She rests a minute at the foot of the stairs under a fluorescent light. Her green silk has parted—she examines her calves, smooth and vast as Jones Beach. How is it her hand can't reach all around her calf? It should—shouldn't it? Should the arms hang to the knees, and should the above-the-waist be as long as the below-the-waist, and how many diamonds between the legs should there be? Her hand—not even both hands will reach around her calf, and her calf is the smallest part of her—except for her ankles and wrists. She wants ice cream.

Who is she? Is she the one who sells thrown-away newspapers on the subway stairs at the Museum of Natural History stop? Her teeth are brown and chipped, her neck puffy, her anklets ripped. She has never been loved by a man; she has never danced for her parents; she doesn't have a daughter on the Scarsdale Track Team. She doesn't lie here feeling herself.

I lie here feeling myself. The whole room rises and falls with Mac's snoring. Where are my own sounds? They take time. No fantasies work. I've learned it's best to feel the presence of no one. To attend to the physical. It's physics. Cold, metallic, miraculous as an eggbeater. It works. When I am good I am very good. The better I am the faster the spokes spin, the less I hear his snoring, the more the spokes blur; the longer this lasts, the harder I cry when the lines reappear. Then the pillow is wet, and I need to get up for a tissue. I must not use this getting up for a tissue as an excuse to get up for something to eat. I must not, but I do.

I open the refrigerator. Leftover potato salad—German style. I don't eat potatoes—I just don't, never have—but I do love to garden through for the green peppers, scallions, celery, and eggs. When I'm done with that I imagine Mac opening the door and finding this poor Irishman's dish; and Kim also, tasting it, examining it, wondering what has gone wrong. It's better to finish it—potatoes and all. Gobble up the evidence. And since I never eat potatoes, if I eat them now, I'm not me. I eat them, but it hasn't worked; I'm still me. I remember the turkey we had for dinner. Mac takes three bites and throws the rest out. I don't dare remind him of the starving children, not with the way I look; so later—now, I scavenge for his bones. There are a few green beans on them, coffee grounds, a piece of cellophane and an eggshell, but nothing that can't be washed off. Why, there's practically a whole meal here—a crime, someone would say. I eat to the bone. I want dessert. Something sweet. I help myself to half a frozen Sara Lee cheesecake and bury the rest, *deep* in the garbage. I want chocolate. We only have unsweetened baking chocolate which tastes like fiberglass but isn't bad with dates and walnuts. I eat all three, in every order, proportion, and combination, and now it's time for the one last thing. I'm trying not to think about the one last thing because we don't have it. We don't have it because with *it* I have absolutely no limit. The closest is nearly ten miles, on the other side of the tracks. The daytime regulars are mostly black, but at night there are all kinds; and at 4 A.M.—why, I imagine at 4 A.M. "John's" is a regular UN. Desperation brings people together. I should hurry, before they run out of my favorite flavors. Now I bet Mac would find that hard to believe—that so many people make runs to "John's" in the middle of the night that you have to drive too fast or they'll run out of your favorite flavors. Mac pretends not to understand desperation, and people never talk about it nowadays. Alpha waves, incest dreams, prostates— yes; desperation—no. But Mac, try to remember. There were nights you'd cry for just one more peanut. I lie, you say. You're right. No scruples. You were strong, you were rigid and free as St. Francis; craving and counting for a few weeks, but once you tapped Mr. Thin Mac on the shoulder, there was no pissing and moaning and only one desire: to free the imprisoned thin Mac. But still, I'm certain you remember—maybe from childhood. Wanting, wanting, wanting. That's how we are, Mac, the junkies at "John's," and more of us than your lean, clean, fart-free body dares to imagine. We nod hello, but never speak, never share opinions on flavors or brands. We have respect. We understand the need to do this thing alone. To take this container to a special, sacred place and do it with a spoon or a fork or without any utensils in whatever manner whatsoever, to be alone, without thought, without edge, to eat. It's an arrangement. We don't mention it; we don't pretend it doesn't exist. But when was the last time you looked anything in the face?—*me*, I think I have no face. I must check; tiptoe down to the mirror in the vestibule—no table or sink there; I can stand up close. I feel my way down the stairs, careful to miss the pictures. There. I turn on the light. A face. I turn my head from side to side—a pale face, it has two eyes with blue puff moons beneath and a nose that leaves a mist and a mouth with cracked lips. When the mouth opens there are teeth. But oh those teeth, Sylvia. Don't you brush your teeth anymore? There are no quarters from the tooth fairy for girls who don't brush. . . . But still there's a face, *hurrah*. I must go wake Mac. He won't mind. Oh, but look. How peaceful he looks. All bones and shadows. This weight loss has

done him good. He looks beautiful. I must not wake him.
Still, I could shake him ever so slightly. He might think he
was dreaming. *Mac. Mac. Look what I've brought you. A
face, a beautiful face.*

—Leslie Lawrence

Revenge

I will get fat.
I will be shaped like a bowl of apples,
globe upon globe.

No more "Hey, baby."
"Hey, fat lady," they'll say.

I will willendorf-waddle across the room,
Lower me into a chair and say "Whew!"
The chair will sigh too.

I will use talcum powder here and there
To keep from chafing.
I will have a house dress.

My sex will disappear in lap-folds;
My eyes will be currants in a white bun-face.

Then *he'll* come back.

"Oh, pardon me. I knew a lady once. Slim—quick—
Smiled easily. Perhaps—?"

Can't help, I'll say.

—Juneil Parmenter

Yesterday and Today

This means nothing to me. Weber-Fechner law. Steven's law. I had breakfast this morning, Granola and coffee. Mechanics of the ear. A "masking" phenomenon is a "white noise" that hides tones of higher frequency. I had breakfast, but as usual I long to be downstairs in a corner of the coffee shop, eating something delicious.

I keep glancing to the right to make sure that guy isn't reading my scribblings. I must keep these personal ramblings out of my lecture notebook. Only Weber-Fechner and the mysteries of the inner ear belong on these pages. On the opposite page is a brave list: 1. Give up coffee. 2. Record dreams. 3. Attend all classes. 4. Exercise every day.

The break. At last, like a cue at the end of a dull sermon (now turn in your hymnbooks and join together . . .), the instructor's voice rises: "Now when we return from the break . . ." The rest is muffled in the rustling and agitated bumping of two hundred bodies. Out of the lecture hall, out, out and down the stairwell to the College Inn.

Here the decor is fake wood and fluorescent light, this tasteless ambience accepted by a single anemic form dangling above the cash register. I half-smile at fellow classmates, but feel distant.

"Hi, Karen!" Can't remember her name.

"Hi." There it is, my sole utterance of the long morning. It hangs like a bubble in front of my face for just an instant, then floats up to pop in the flickering white light. Gone.

I'm not really hungry. Coffee and . . .

I'm not really hungry, waiting in line. The teacher's assistant purchases a modest can of grapefruit juice, and exits, holding his treasure carefully. Voices, laughter. Most students ask for coffee, then lean eagerly over the doughnut tray.

There they are, not discreetly hidden in a pink box, not enclosed in a glass showcase, but brazenly exhibited within reach of every customer. Glistening, voluptuous doughnuts. I want the biggest, largest, most chocolate-covered sugar-glazed cream-filled.

I make it out the door with coffee and a plain old-fashioned. My father always said, "If you're fat, just push yourself away from the table. It's just a matter of *willpower.*" Climbing the steps with enormous regret, I ruminate about what sort of a pathetic organ my will might be. Perhaps I can exercise it by intoning these magical words with each step: Willpower. Fortitude. Moral fiber. Resolution.

Yesterday I bought two of the biggest most everything, guaranteed to please and to induce stomachache and tooth decay. I ate one on the way upstairs, hiding number two in my purse to be eaten during the lecture. And yesterday I returned downstairs after class for a bagel with cream cheese—stale, but I ate it nonetheless, on the bus into town. There I bought two scoops of ice cream (one fudge nut and one coffee), and a bag of assorted cookies from the bakery (dry and tasteless), and a dish of strawberry frozen yogurt, and ingested them all with quick bites and swallows of mechanical deliberation, while wandering down the crowded street. Ostensibly window-shopping, but actually eating eating eating.

Yesterday was a bad day. I recall moving slowly through the housewives and tourists, watching people from under heavy brows. The warm spring atmosphere was shimmering unpleasantly. I had felt queasy and faint, because I had consumed as much food as my stomach could bear, and then I had thrown up in the blue-tiled rest room in Macy's.

After I had heaved it all up, I blew my nose and wiped the toilet rim. (Such a good girl; I always clean up after myself.) I held my head for a minute. Something was building inside me, something—What was it—hate, grief, disappointment? They were all just words to me, and out I strolled into the bright sunlight. Window-shopping. Don't hate yourself, I told my faint reflection. Look at the pretty dresses and don't think.

And now the professor has returned to his pulpit, and now my classmates dutifully reenter the large dark hall. But I hesitate halfway back and sit down on the steps, a lost sheep. I bend over my notebook and write this: I want to eat. I want doughnuts and ice cream and macaroni salad, and a deli sandwich and carrot cake, and chocolate. I want it all, everything. I want to feed myself.

Then I draw a deep breath and lean back to think. Why do I want to eat when I'm not hungry? What does the sensation of hunger mean to me? It feels like emptiness, needing, feeling. Too much feeling.

Yesterday I walked aimlessly up and down the shopping mall and thought about all the other bad days. My temples were pulsing an insistent rhythm, and I found it difficult to meet the eyes of other people. Especially men's eyes. One man sprawled on a bench eyed me up and down and up again with a belligerent gleam. (My mother said, "Always hold your stomach in when boys are around.") I stared blankly back at him, through him.

"Hello!" he challenged. I passed by with stiff steps.

"Nice ass!"

I glanced back at him. "Yours would be pretty cute too if your head wasn't up it," I retaliated without breaking stride.

"What? Well, fuck you!" (Just keep walking. Walk; don't look back.)

That was yesterday, or was it Tuesday? Today, writing down my thoughts seems to help somehow. Tapping the inner ear. Am I hungry? (What would my shrink say—are you really hungry?) I've forgotten what hunger is like. My shrink would advise me to go home and do something *really* nurturing, emotionally nourishing, or to express these pent-up feelings. Stamp around in my room, yell into the mattress, chew on my pillow.

Then perhaps I wouldn't be so jumpy. Then I could water my plants and stroke my cat. I shut my eyes and see my big black cat dozing on the balcony. If only I could be a lazy stupid feline, nothing to worry me on a fine morning like this aside from small clouds and a few ear mites. In the A.M. she sunbathes; in the afternoon she retires indoors to the windowsill. For her the long hours slip by uncounted, into evening shadows; she patiently keeps watch at the window. Children running; the mail truck stopping, starting; a sudden rustling of leaves. If only I could gain some peace of mind. That would be everything to me.

—Lisa Wagner

The Joy of Self-Indulgence

I didn't actually start wearing Chubbettes until I was in the third grade. At the time, of course, I was too young to know it, but Chubbette was the result of some pretty weird things that had started happening before kindergarten. I'd begun to hear voices.

The first time I noticed them was late one night after I'd watched *Lassie Come Home*. Or maybe it was an old Dorothy Lamour movie—I don't remember which. Anyway, there I was, lying in bed and thinking about how popular Donna Gill was and all . . . when, suddenly, they were just there. Not my imagination or anything dumb like that, but real words that glommed onto me like household cement.

Avocado sandwich.

Now, I don't know about you, but when I hear something like that I can't just ignore it. I figure my body's trying to tell me something. Like maybe I have iron-poor blood. Or maybe one day, if I'm not careful, I'll wake up and all my teeth will have fallen out. So, I'll tell you straight out, when my body talks I listen. And if it says it needs an avocado sandwich, that's just what it gets.

Anyway, that's how I got mixed up with this Chubbette business.

Later, though, when I grew up and got into high school, I really started getting worked up about it—I mean, about wearing Chubbettes. I noticed, for instance, that none of the girls who went out with football players wore Chubbettes. They wore body suits and thin, swirly skirts and stacked heels. I knew Donna Gill didn't wear them because she told me so in P.E. She was a size 9 junior petite. In fact, the only other girl I knew who wore Chubbettes was Sally McCreedy—and she dropped out of school for a month and came back real skinny.

So there I was, the only girl in all of South Franklin High who wore Chubbettes, except for Fat Wanda who hung out in the bathroom, and she didn't count.

Then one day I started getting what you might call revelations. Like, I was eating lunch with this brainy type Jeremy Huston who was always spouting off about economic theory when suddenly I looked down to find that his theory had been put into practice. I was the victim of spiraling inflation. My zipper had just popped.

Now, I know there are a lot worse things in life than a busted zipper, but when you're in high school, stuff like that can really destroy you. So I got up real casual and bought a third pack of cashews—you know, as sort of a cover-up—then ran real fast to the girls' gym to change into my monkey suit. That's when things *really* started getting strange.

Like, when I walked into Psych class, no one noticed. And, I mean, people notice when you wear your gym suit to class. I guess they figure you got your period or something. Anyway, everybody just kept talking like I was Cosmo Topper's ghost, so I opened up my cashews and checked out the blackboard.

That's when I got Revelation Number Two. Topic for the day: SUBSTITUTION.

At first, of course, I figured the teacher was sick and that we'd get to goof off for a while. Then I found out they were talking about crazy people, so I tuned in like I did to Wolfman Jack.

What they do is try this SUBSTITUTION thing on loonies.

I guess it costs too much to keep them locked up all the time. It's like the ones with real weird phobias try to get phobias that aren't quite so weird, and if it works, everything's supposed to turn out okay.

Well, you can imagine what I thought of SUBSTITUTION. I mean, the idea started to bubble up in me like peroxide. So I asked Jeremy Huston to look it up in his dad's *Psychological Dictionary,* and he quoted what he found from his binder the next day.

Substitution: The replacement of one goal with another when the individual's route to the first has been blocked.

Let me tell you, there's no bigger block than popping the zipper in your last Chubbette.

I don't remember exactly when I found The Substitute. It could have been that day or maybe a month later. All I remember are the pictures.

The first one I saw one night while I was munching buttered popcorn and staring at the tube. I got a feeling someone was watching me. So when the commercial came on, I looked down . . . and, sure enough, there was this lady on the back of a magazine staring up at me like the Mona Lisa.

Now, let's get this straight. This was no ordinary lady. I mean, she had *class,* like Dorothy Lamour—thin and real nice ankles. And I could tell right off she didn't eat avocados, although she may have used them on her face.

So, there she was, lounging on this picnic bench with ferns and stuff all around, while this strong Dan Rather type stroked the bottom of her foot with a pine needle. I zoomed right in on that . . . and there, in the very center of the picture, was the key.

This woman, like my mother (who looked nothing like her), smoked cigarettes.

At first, of course, it was revolting. I mean, I can still remember the time we drove to Lone Pine when my mother lit up with all the windows closed and I threw up out the windwing. She was always puffing on those things: when she got out of bed, when she got into bed, when she sat on the john, when she made egg noodles.

But when I really got to studying that picture, I thought it was sexy. I mean, just the way she held it. So I cut it out and took it in to my English teacher the next day and said, "How would you describe that?"

"Languid," she said. "Definitely languid."

Never in my life had a word sounded so beautiful.

About a week later I saw the other picture. It was on the back of one of my father's books. This is how I remember my father: smelly socks bordering the rim of the wastebasket beside his bed, and, above them, on the table, a book by Mark Twain. Anyway, there he was—Twain, I mean—and why hadn't I noticed it before? There was cigarette smoke sneaking out from underneath his moustache.

What more can I say? Ten minutes later, in front of my bedroom mirror, I took up smoking.

It didn't take long for me to learn that you don't just "take up" smoking. Like jogging, it demands a lot of willpower, not to mention stamina.

For one thing, you have to get to the place where inhaling doesn't make you barf in the toilet. Then you have to get to where the cigarette looks like it *belongs* in your hand and isn't just stuck there like a kite in a tree.

There's an etiquette to smoking—rules with fine lines that are just as valid as which fork to use on your salad. For instance, you wouldn't want to smoke with Fat Wanda until you knew how to inhale. In fact, you probably wouldn't smoke with her at all unless you could blow smoke rings—though they could never, of course, be quite like hers.

It was beautiful, the way she did it. I mean, almost like ballet. She'd squat down beneath the sanitary napkin dispenser, tilt back her head, and work her mouth like she was going to sing Handel's *Messiah*. Then, out they'd come . . . a perfect trail of rings that would expand and float like voile up to the skylight.

I asked her once just how she did that. She said a person had to have *élan*.

Six months later, I boxed up my Chubbettes and donated them to the church rummage sale. My smoke rings that day were like carrier pigeons sending up little messages of joy.

By the time I graduated I was blowing rings around Fat Wanda. I mean, I could smoke more cigarettes than Twain could have stashed on a barge. In fact, as the years passed, I got so good that when I married Howard, the priest said, "You may exchange your smoke rings now."

I think that's where I goofed—I mean, getting married. Because just a few months after that, I started getting congested . . . and then a few months after that, I came down with insomnia. On account of my coughing.

One night while I was just coughing away, I thought of this dumb book we'd had to read in high school. The main character was always "hawking phlegm." Now, I don't know about you, but I think those have got to be the two grossest words in the English language. So I got up and figured I'd better rethink this SUBSTITUTION thing.

I think I thought about it for exactly five minutes. I

mean, "élan" and "languid" are nothing compared to "hawking phlegm." So I wound up flushing my cigarettes, one at a time, down the toilet, until it overflowed.

That's about the time they came back. The voices, I mean. There, at three in the morning, while I was standing in a pool of soggy butts, I heard them. No doubt about it.

Avocado sandwich.

Of course we were out of avocados, but I'd had plenty of time to perfect the art of SUBSTITUTION. I just fixed a stack of BLTs. No sweat.

Then I got to thinking about what my Psych teacher would say. And, I mean, I could almost hear his voice. He'd say you don't just "quit" smoking. He'd say you have to plan for it, and he'd use words like "mature," "rational," and "meeting the challenge."

For instance (he'd say), you wouldn't want to quit the same day your septic tank caved in. Ideally, you'd pick a good time in your life; e.g., great job, terrific marriage, plenty of money to pay the bills, no hassles, no kids. Right. You'd find "creative substitutes" (besides eating). And when you'd exhausted all the alternatives and found you were still fighting the urge to light up, you'd give it the ole karate chop and then reward yourself for your victory. For instance, maybe you'd eat.

Me, I started out biting my fingernails (that is, after I ate the BLTs). I cleaned out the kitchen cabinets. You know . . . ate up the peanuts, the baking chocolate, the marshmallows, the box of stale crackers I'd been meaning to throw out.

Then I figured sure enough I was heading for Chubbettes again, so I took up jogging. Which was fine until I got blisters. So then I took up writing, figuring that's how a person vents frustration.

Howard came home one night and found me waiting for him right at the door. "Who died?"

"Nobody." I waved a stack of papers at him. (Actually, I'd written only one page, but I figured the rest would make a good impression.)

"You *wrote* something?" He kicked back in the recliner and lit a cigarette. "That's great, Rennie! Let's hear it."

"Okay," I said, "but you have to understand this is *haiku*. Are you in the right place for that?"

He slapped the arms of his chair. So I stood in front of him the way Jeremy Huston did the time he spoke to the Kiwanis on "Let's Clean Up America," and recited the day's work:

> Chewing and gnashing
> sends another piece of food
> down the hatch again.

Howard looked at me sort of funny, so I decided to brush the potato chip crumbs off my jeans.

He just shook his head and said, "Oh, God, Rennie."

The voices were no longer stopping at avocados. Now they wanted ham-and-walnut appetizers, homemade doughnuts, cherries and whipped cream and all that good stuff. I started looking to see what other "mature" and "rational" adults did. I mean, besides eat and smoke.

My neighbor, I learned, brushes crumbs. Even when there aren't any crumbs she brushes crumbs and talks about her poor sister Isabel.

"Always picking her face," she said, brushing joyfully. "Isn't it sad how some people never seem to solve their problems?"

"It certainly is," I said, and politely excused myself. I ran home to pick my face.

While I was standing in front of the bathroom mirror, I heard this strange sound . . . like a leaky faucet dripping on a sponge. So, I checked out the shower and found my cat Leonard. He was happily engrossed in the task of sucking his leg. (A classic symptom, according to my Psych teacher. Weaned too early.)

I phoned a psychiatrist. "Look, I have this problem."

"Oh?"

"I don't want to suck my leg."

Her voice strained for objectivity. "I see."

"And I've been . . . well . . . hearing voices."

Her voice changed then. She sounded like she'd just been told she had a winning sweepstakes ticket. "Oh, this is *very* interesting; do go on. I want to hear *all* about it."

"Uh . . . you'll have to excuse me. I think I hear my mother calling."

Now that was really strange, because she did call about five minutes later.

"Well, hello dear! And what are *you* having for dinner?" My mother always says that on the phone. She says that way you play it safe. *Everybody* likes to talk about food.

"Chicken-filled pastry boats."

"Sounds yummy," she said.

"They were."

Her voice took on its "confider" tone then. "Out with it, Rennie. What's eating you?"

"It's not so much what's eating me," I said. "It's more like what I'm eating."

"Don't tell me. Let me guess. You quit smoking."

I swear, my mother was born with a crystal ball in her hand.

"Look, Rennie," she continued, "do you remember your Uncle Harold?"

"Sure." How could I forget? "Had three wives and joined the circus."

"No, no, that was Clifford. Harold's the one who quit smoking and turned alcoholic."

That's when I hung up on her.

I dove for Howard's cigarettes.

For a while, just for old time's sake, I puffed languidly and blew a couple of smoke rings. (And I mean they had class, like Fat Wanda's: cool and light and breezy.) Then for some dumb reason I started hearing voices again. Only this time they were the words of Jeremy Huston.

"You can cure the smog problem, but then you have inflation." (Check.) "You can stop inflation, but then you have recession." (Check.) "But then," he'd say, "that's when you *really* have problems." (Double check.)

Well, me, I'm not into having problems. I've decided I'm just not cut out for wearing Chubbettes, picking my face, or crumb-brushing. In fact, even avocados don't thrill me like they used to. So, I smoke. No big deal. Just weaned too early, I guess.

I *have* solved the problem of hawking phlegm, though— and that's all I really wanted to do in the first place. From here on out, I plan to do just like Twain did: I refuse to smoke more than one cigarette at a time.

—Joan P. Campbell

Devil Sweet

You are a magnet.
You disguise yourself
As a lifeline,
Yet I know you
To be my destruction.
I move toward you
Even as I strain
To avoid your field.
Struggling free,
I remain haunted
By your palate stroke;
And energy moves me
Toward you once more.
Then as tongue rejoices,
Head sighs
And wonders
If death has won
Another round.

—*Micki Seltzer*

My Hunger Has a Name*

My hunger has a name; it has a face, a personality of its own. My hunger is a child who lives inside me. I call my hunger Molly. Around her small body, I've grown longer, developed breasts, a woman's face. But she is the beginning.

When I close my eyes, I see her clearly: she is five or six years old, thin and wraithlike. Her hair is brown, uncombed and stringy. Her mouth remains open, wanting, and her hands reach out, pleading. She cries one word, like a doll that you turn upside down, and this she repeats over and over. Mama. Mama.

Molly's mother has arms and legs slender as cigarettes, a face as beautiful as a model's but unfinished, as if an artist forgot her flesh when he was drawing her, leaving slashes for cheekbones, jaw and forehead. Her hair, streaked in sunbursts by the beautician's hand, is pulled away from her face and piled in back with the help of a modified wig ("Nun's hair," her mother calls it). From the front, the effect is startling: her hair stands five inches above her forehead before it sweeps to the french knot in back. Hair spray holds the effect in place.

From the age of four, Molly senses her mother's discontent and tunes herself to the scale of her moods. When she hears ugly words between her parents, her nerves vibrate at higher and higher frequencies until it seems like her bones are shattering when dishes are broken, doors slammed. Molly is terrified

*Special thanks to June Brindel and the women in our section for their help with this piece.

of the rage she witnesses: Will her mother leave? Will her father? What then? How could she live?

Panicked by the possibilities, she takes it upon herself to make her mother happy. She will speak sweetly, she will never complain. She will be there always. She will be everything her father is not. Her father, it seems, can care for himself. He doesn't cry, calls her "pussycat" and comforts her when she is punished. He leaves for work before Molly is awake and returns after she is asleep.

Each day, Molly reads her mother's face, searching for a sign that will tell her what she must do, say, be that day to make her smile. Her goal is to become an expert in the language of her mother; to know the meaning of each tone, fleeting glance, body movement—and then, to know how to translate them. Some days, she does it well and her mother calls her "darling." Other days it backfires and she is yelled at, or worse, cornered by the dreaded rage and hit. Then, she returns to her room and sobs. Not from the physical pain, but from the knowledge that she is losing her mother.

When she is fourteen, they move to a larger house. Molly hears her mother talking on the phone late at night. Her father, at work or in bed, does not hear. Molly's mother murmurs on the phone, whispers in words soft as a bird's breast, says "I love you." Molly can sense that it is to a man that she coos. She feels nauseated. She tries to imagine her mother with another man. What does he look like? Does she lay naked with him? Where do they "do it"? How *could* she? Molly feels betrayed, helpless and in more pain than she has ever known.

She writes her mother notes: "You are breaking the commandment that says, 'Thou shalt not commit adultery.' You are a liar. You are a cheat. I hate you" but she never sends them. She wants to believe that she is wrong, that she is imagining things and tomorrow she will find it has been a bad dream. Besides, though she is angry, she realizes that if she is to keep her mother, she has to fight harder than ever and that means she cannot confront her with the truth.

Molly tells no one her secret. When she talks about her family, she lies. She pretends that she is Kitten on "Father Knows Best" and that they eat mashed potatoes and meat loaf together at night, instead of the Swanson's frozen dinners she fixes for herself and eats alone.

Molly's mother develops a schedule. She leaves the house sometime in the afternoon and doesn't return until 4 or 5 A.M. Sometimes she doesn't come home at all. When Molly, pretending innocence, asks her father, "Where's Mom?" he mumbles an excuse: she stayed at Lil's or Bobbie's or Fran's. It was too late to drive home, he says. She tries not to think about why he doesn't know, or isn't speaking, the truth.

Molly, too, develops a schedule. After her mother leaves, she wanders from room to room in a veil of tears. She does not know what to do with herself in the empty house. Soon she discovers an ally: food. She knows how concerned her mother is with thinness, her own and Molly's, so she eats. And eats. She sneaks candy, cookies, ice cream into her room, even when no one is home. Food becomes her solace; it never goes away. Fat becomes her nemesis: it is her weight, she reasons, that drives her mother away.

The ringing of the phone startles me as I sit now, writing. "Hello?" "Hi sweetheart." "Hi Mom." We chat about my cousin, the weather in New York, the weather here and then she tells me that she can't come to visit as we had planned; something else has come up. Tears form in my throat. I ask her what is so important, tell her I am hurt about her priorities. She says it is finances, she hopes I will understand, she loves me. I tell her I don't want to talk anymore and hang up.

Molly takes over. I cry, wander into the living room, lay down on the floor and cry again. It is that same half acre of pain: I want her to love me, to want me, why doesn't she?

What's *wrong* with me? I think about eating, open the refrigerator door, close it again. I feel like the earth after a volcanic eruption: charred and desolate.

"I *did* love you," she once said, when I told her about the hunger of those years, "but I couldn't stay in the house. I felt like a caged animal. I was crazed. All I could think of was myself. It had nothing to do with you. . . ."

Fragments of conversations we've had: my mother as a little girl, fat and lonely. Her parents at work, she'd return from school and sit at the kitchen table, eating. "I tried for years to get my mother's attention," she told me, "but no matter what I did, she didn't seem to notice. My sister was always prettier and thinner. When we grew up and *I* got thinner and richer, my sister was in trouble, so my mother still focused on her. Always on her." She once told me she knew soon after she married my father that she wanted a divorce, but her mother got down on her hands and knees and pleaded with her to stay. "I wanted to please her so badly," she said, "so I stayed."

My mother has a Molly.

When I think of her eating alone in her shabby Bronx apartment, and me eating alone in our big fancy house, I cry for us both: generation after generation of hungry women.

Images of her now: hair cropped close to her face, arms and legs in soft curves, a satisfied face. I think of the ritual bubble baths we take whenever we are together now, talking until the water gets cold. In the sixties when everyone was smoking pot, she wanted to try it. When she saw furry animals walking off the wallpaper, we laughed till we cried. She's managed to fly with me through my twenties, always interested in why I was doing a particular thing, what I was learning. She followed my journey from India through vegetarianism to African dance; she's meditated, cooks brown rice and tofu and knows how to rock her pelvis. "You are my best teacher," she's told me many times, "and I feel very lucky."

*   *   *

Lying on the living room floor, I realize I am still expecting her to fill the hungry spaces. I can accept her only if I am willing to accept her limitations and give up on the dream of a perfect mother. When I let go of the dream, the focus immediately changes from anguishing about the ways she *doesn't* love me to appreciating the ways she *does*. I don't really want to give up this fantasy of perfect mother love; it's so comforting. But it also leaves me powerless because of the dependence it creates on another person, a person with a Molly of her own.

Accepting my mother means that I stop looking at her through Molly's eyes.

Something else has become clear to me: by trying to be lover/partner/friend to my mother, I set myself up for disappointment. As a child needing her love, I could not possibly be a partner giving her love. Yet it was upon her acceptance of me as that partner that I judged myself a failure or success. Consequently, I felt like a failure—unloved and unwanted—most of the time. It *is* possible that she loved me as a mother loves a child, but intent as I was on being her partner, I would have missed those signs. Hunger is so focused on what it is not getting and on its own definition of love and fulfillment that it often misses the very nourishment it is crying for.

Molly returns. Her presence is a reminder that during those years of trying to be an adult, I lost a childhood. Somewhere, in the wild flapping of wings, I forgot how to play, how to shout at summer. My mind was always on my mother, even when I was climbing a tree or touching the underside of a frog's belly.

Molly's hunger was also for her *own* attention. Her hunger was for herself. And she's still very sad about those years.

I tell her it's okay to be sad, it was a loss, and we both grieve for that.

But it's not too late. There are still sparkling days and treehouses, falling stars and merry-go-rounds. Cinderella hasn't grown up and Bambi is still in the forest. I'll invite Molly to come giggle with my friend Sara and me during one of those afternoons when we throw all the clothes out of the closet and play dress-up. Or she can push Howard into the lake and dissolve into laughter because he has all his clothes on. Or she can stick her used gum under the table where someone will find it or hand out chocolate-covered ants to the women in my groups.

I can tell that Molly likes these ideas because she does something she's never done before. She smiles.

Eating as Metaphor, Part 2: NOURISHMENT

"On a physical level food is nourishment and on an emotional level food is nourishment."

—a Breaking Free workshop participant

Nourishment

To nourish means to comfort; to cherish, to support; a dictionary adds "to supply with matter necessary for growth."

Nourishment is specific; what nourishes you in one situation may not nourish you in another. Nourishment is personal; what nourishes another may not nourish you. The type of nourishment you choose is dependent on the way you interpret your hunger. If you are unwilling to allow yourself to be hungry, you shut out the possibility of nourishing yourself. If you can't hear your needs, you can't fulfill them. The quality of your life is dependent on the ways you nourish yourself.

A woman in a workshop told me, "On a physical level, food is nourishment; and on an emotional level, food is nourishment." She laughed and I laughed, but since she was thirty pounds overweight and in a marriage she'd rather have been out of, we both knew she meant what she said. She uses food as her support, her comfort, her sole source of nourishment.

If you use food or any other tangible substance—alcohol, cigarettes, drugs—as your main source of psychic "nourishment," you never get full. Food, being a tangible substance, cannot satisfy intangible needs. It can numb you, drug you, but it cannot nourish you.

Your chest aches. You're not sure why, but you know that it hurts, and it's uncomfortable to hurt. You want to do something about it quickly; you want the pain to go away. So you eat the ice cream in the refrigerator; and for a while the ache freezes over, but it doesn't dissolve. You push it into the background: you focus your attention on the chocolate chips sliding down your throat; and afterwards, the glaze of a full stomach puts you to sleep. In the morning you awaken with stomach pains and a dull ache in your chest. No ice cream left. Today it's potato chips or cookies or candy or anything in the refrigerator: cold vegetables, frozen cake, fingerfuls of peanut butter. But the hurt remains. The ache—and what caused it—moves deeper into your body, curling around your heart, settling in your bones. The food has not touched it.

Watching a child try to put a round peg in a square hole, you know it is useless. Yet the futility of using food for psychic nourishment is not as obvious. You eat but you remain forever hungry—full but hungry. At twenty, fifty, one hundred pounds overweight, you are undernourished.

Food satisfies when the hunger is physical, and only then can it be considered nourishment. Every other time you "use" food, you leave yourself. You walk out the door and leave yourself starving. You wouldn't leave your best friend in time of need. You wouldn't even leave an acquaintance. But you leave yourself over and over. And each time it happens, you come a little closer to true starvation.

Every time you reach for food when you're not hungry, you are getting a signal of need. If you recognize that, you're lucky; you've found a way of getting your own attention. Some people never realize the access they have to their inner lives. Some people become so cut off from their bodies and so attuned to everyone else's needs, judgments, and demands that they ignore their own. They learn how to nourish their spouses, children, friends, but they don't take time to learn to feed themselves.

At least you have an avenue into your inner world. Your compulsive eating can become a sign that you need something— even though you don't know what it is or how to get it. Rather than viewing it as a seizure that overtakes and propels you toward food, you can use it as an indicator, a barometer of your nonphysical hunger. You don't have to eat because you want to eat; you don't have to reach for the ice cream because it has suddenly become all you can think about. At that very moment—when you know you want to eat but you also know you are not hungry—you are giving yourself the message that some support, some comfort, some cherishing is needed. The drive to eat compulsively is not an uncontrollable instinct; it is a cry for help.

If you truly understand this about your compulsive eating, you can release yourself from the craziness by which you have defined it; you can stop beating yourself up. You can consider yourself fortunate to be getting a message that is so easy to read, and you can begin to explore alternate nourishments.

The path between sensing you are in need of something and reaching for food to satisfy it is well grooved and automatic. You don't think about it anymore. You are bored and so you eat. You hurt and so you eat. By now it is the easiest path to follow, because it requires no effort. It has become a habit. It also takes you, albeit momentarily, to where you want to go: out of the emotional discomfort. There are other ways, however, to knock yourself out if that's what you want to do. You can sleep, go to a movie, watch TV. You can play with a child (a dog, a cat), sing to a bird, read a trashy novel. You can distract yourself without having to face waking up in the morning sick to your stomach.

Nourishment is specific; what comforts you one day might disturb you the next. Sometimes knocking yourself out is what you need; sometimes the situation demands to be handled. A confrontation may be needed; or a good cry might work to relieve your anxiety more than your favorite candy bar. Nourishment takes time; figuring out what you need is not so simple as going to the grocery store. You've got to feel that you're worth your own time. Are you important enough to be listened to? Are you worthy of your own attention? Are your needs just as important as your mother's? Your lover's? Your children's? Or are you going to continue smothering yourself with food? Is eating, drinking, smoking your only way out? Do you have to die to get what you want?

Lilly Penn was a typical Jewish grandmother. She made luscious blintzes, chopped liver and borscht. She turned her back on any boyfriend of mine who wasn't Jewish, turned off her hearing aid when she wasn't interested in the conversation, and spoke Yiddish fluently, especially when she didn't want me to know what she was saying. She was like a bull: tough, resilient, outspoken. Everyone thought she would live to be a hundred. Except for one thing: she didn't pay attention to her own needs. She spent years catering to her children and, when they left, to her husband. Clucking around him endlessly, she grew fat on her own food. He became a picky, irritable old man who demanded that every one of his desires be met immediately; she obeyed. When she got cancer of the uterus and had to stay in bed, he complained, he yelled, he fussed. Where were his eggs cooked exactly three and one-half minutes? The coffee cake? The butter cookies for dessert? Why couldn't she get up and fix him dinner, wash his shorts? She had created a monster, and she knew it. She grew pale and wan, and her voice became as thin as antique lace.

After admitting herself in to the hospital for the third time, she told the nurse she didn't want to go home to her husband again. "I should have divorced him thirty years ago," she told my mother. But at eighty-two, what could she do? What options were open to her? Only one that she could see clearly—death. So the tough old lady made her graceful exit, leaving her fragile, fussy husband to fend for himself.

The essential question is: Will you feed yourself with "matters necessary for growth," or will you continue to ignore your needs, killing yourself slowly with food or drink? Will you nourish yourself or won't you?

A fundamental beginning to the process of nourishing yourself is giving yourself permission to do so. For many women, the thought of taking time for themselves is foreign. Their days are spent watching over their brood of children, their friends, their partners. And then, when the well is dry, they eat for replenishment; they eat for strength. It is no accident that ninety percent of compulsive eaters are women. These women get from food what they give to others: an inexhaustible supply of energy. Yet it is these same women who populate diet centers, buy diet books, keep diet doctors in business.

If you walk around with a constant gnawing, with a body that is always empty and always full, food is not working for you. You are undernourished. And if you yourself are not nourished, then the quality of what you give others is only a thin echo of what it could be.

Ask yourself what nourishes you. Not what is fastest but what fully satisfies that longing, that craving for attention. A bubble bath? A nap in the afternoon? Do you ever allow yourself to sit down for half an hour with nothing to do, nowhere to go?

When I first tell people to make a list of ways in which to nourish themselves without food, they stare at me blankly. "There is nothing else," someone told me last night; "at least nothing else that is so immediately gratifying as food." What she didn't say was that turning to food was ultimately so *un*gratifying that she had joined a group to break free of it.

If you've been using food to quiet the voice of hunger for many years, it will take time and patience to discover the subtle intonations, the inflections of that hungry voice. A few steps before you reach for food is another, more satisfying alternative: a quiet time, a walk, an intimate conversation, a touch. But in order to hear the possibilities, you must care about yourself enough to listen. You must feel that there is a level to your hunger that you are capable of finding.

Most compulsive eaters see themselves as bottomless. They believe that they can never get enough food, attention or love. And in fact, if you use food for a hunger that is not physical, it is true: you can never get enough. After a binge of three gallons of ice cream, a large pizza and two packages of cookies, that which was hungry remains hungry.

To nourish yourself, you must believe in yourself, believe that you are worth nurturing. You must learn to read your own needs, rather than pretend that what nurtures someone else also nurtures you. This means being willing to be authentic, true to an inner clarity that is waiting to speak when you are ready to listen. You must be willing to unfold yourself until you get to the quintessence that is you.

In *New Age Magazine* (Vol. 75), Dr. Bernie Siegel, a cancer specialist at Yale University Hospital, says: "Most people get sick because they're not living their own lives. They are living the roles that everyone else imposes upon them, and they don't know enough to say the help I need is mental. The disease is a message to take a new road in your life."

The place to start, he feels, is by loving yourself. "I believe that when you abuse yourself, you abuse the world, in a sense. But if you learn to love yourself, you become an expert in self-preservation. You become an expert in your own healing. You begin to bloom, and then the whole world blooms around you."

Cancer is not compulsive eating, but Dr. Siegel's views are not inapplicable here. Allow yourself to be nourished.

Bloom.

The Double-Edged Gift

I.

At 1A.M. Bernie and Thelma Kemfert walked across the Racquet Club parking lot toward their car. They were the last couple to leave Friday Night Mixed Doubles, a club event which offered the members a chance to drink too much and to cultivate a fantasy about an affair. Watching her feet, Thelma moved quickly. She reached her side of the car and waited by the locked door, hugging her shivering body. The clear desert air in the empty lot magnified the noises her husband made as he shambled through the gravel, humming the song he'd heard in the bar, mumbling something about "paradise" every few seconds. He stared at his feet, flapping his outstretched arms as he tried to place one foot in front of the other to walk a straight line. Thelma watched, a rush of hatred surging through her. The vision of Bernie bumbling across the dance floor clutching the curvaceous body of a young girl to him erased the compassion Thelma would normally have felt for his current condition. The public humiliation she had suffered scooped her hollow. To keep from crying, she muttered to herself, "Look at him, totally ignoring me, unaware of the pain I feel because he fondled that girl on the dance floor." Angered by his insensitivity, she called, "Bern," but the sound of her petulant wail made her regret the impulsive behavior. At least she could conduct herself with dignity, could rise above this debasement.

"Yeah." He looked toward her and teetered, catching himself against the trunk of the car. "Oh, yeah, yeah. Sorry, Thel." He steadied himself on the car as he walked toward her. While he fumbled at the lock, she stood behind him breathing his smell of cigars and whiskey. "Didn't mean to neglect you, Thel."

"Oh, I'm used to it. After tonight, I . . ." She stopped, sensing that tears were inevitable if she continued to speak. She gnawed at the inside of her mouth, hating her lack of control.

Bernie peered over his shoulder at her. "Now, what the hell do you mean?"

She felt his eyes on her. She sighed and turned her face from him. He was going to assume he was blameless. Her eyes burned.

He turned the key in the lock. "Ah, shit. I have a few drinks, dance a couple of dances, and you get pissed."

On the seven-mile drive home, he sang along with the radio turned to a volume that hurt her ears. She stared at the night landscape flashing through the blur of her tears and pressed her fingers about her forearms to keep herself from visibly trembling. If he looked her way, she didn't want him to see her crying. When he ran through a yellow light turning red, she involuntarily jammed her foot on the floor to brake the car. Relaxing her leg, she considered the irony of the subconscious mind. At the moment, she didn't care whether she lived or died.

She locked herself in the bathroom, took an extra-long shower, brushed her teeth, and stared at her face in the mirror as she massaged night cream into her wrinkles. If she delayed long enough, she could avoid speaking to Bernie; he'd be sleeping when she crawled in beside him.

The reading light beside the bed was dim. Bernie was lying on his back. As she approached, Thelma saw that his eyes were open. She'd turned the bathroom light off. To return to the bathroom to avoid the confrontation would be too obvious. She sat on the bed with her back to him. "Thel." He reached across the bed, tracing a finger along the small of her back. She stiffened. The audacity of the man. Could he really believe she would gratefully fall into his arms? Kiss and make up? She shuddered.

"Ah, hell." He flopped over on his side, muttering into his pillow, and switched off the light. Within minutes he was snoring.

Lying next to Bern, she felt sucked empty—from the top of her head, through her mouth, down her throat, past her belly, into her guts. Her body was a hollow black shell. Her head throbbed. He called it dancing. Dear God, just dancing. He had held that girl for hours, pressing her beautiful young body against his, listening to her talk with an attentiveness that Thelma could never even remember having been granted. Maybe ten years ago during their brief courtship; she couldn't remember. She'd been continually amazed because a man liked her, sought her company; she had felt as if she were holding her breath, reminding herself not to hope for too much, not to expect a thing so she wouldn't get hurt. When he asked her to marry him, all she could think was, Somebody wants me; somebody wants to marry me. Perhaps it wasn't love, whatever that was. He had wanted her and that was enough. But she was a fool: fat and ugly and foolish. Obviously, wanting was not enough. She brushed her eyelids closed with the fingers of one hand and rested her forearm across her eyes as if to hold them shut so she could drift into sleep.

Maybe he had been seeing the girl before tonight. Maybe it was an affair. What contempt he must feel. Right in front of her he had practically devoured the girl, then brushed it off as nothing and assumed that Thelma would sleep with him. Life without Bernie—what would it be? He was everything. She'd done everything he ever wanted: worked and handed over the paycheck because he "knew how to manage," never had children because— well, because—because she had such a strange body it couldn't produce children—but they'd never gone ahead with adoption because of Bernie, because Bernie always said, "We're so happy without kids." She'd waited on him because he hated housework. She'd let him make all the decisions because he knew best. Even her obses- sion with Overeaters Anonymous, which had replaced her obsession with eating, was really for him. He liked slender women, not dowdy frumps like Thelma. For six weeks she had followed the O.A. food plan by weighing and measuring the food for her meals; she chewed sugarless gum so violently it made her jaws ache, gnawed on her fingers until her cuticles bled, called fellow mem- bers when she was so desperate that she knew she'd begin eating again. She had lived each day as if it would be her last on abstinence. She knew she suffered from a disease. If she tasted the wrong food, she would begin to eat wildly, stuffing herself until she was ill. To care for herself, she had become an apothecary, choosing foods and preparing them with their medicinal properties in mind. Consumption of the proper balance at the proper time could keep her disease under control. Learning to live without the drug of food was hell. She had denied herself the comfort, the friendship of food. The only way she'd been able to do it was by promising herself it was only for a day that she'd go without food, only for today. And what had it mattered? Why had she denied herself? She had given her life away, and what'd she gotten? Nothing. He saw her as nothing: a thing to be used and thrown away. She wished she'd cried. Not so he'd see her, but so she wouldn't feel this empty, empty aching. If she could stop this physical pain—go to sleep— Sleep could move her from this pain for now. Sleeping pills might block the feeling. Maybe some aspirin. She got up and felt her way through the dark to the medicine cabinet.

At 4 A.M. she decided a glass of wine might help. She'd tried everything to bring the smothering blanket of sleep, and the harder she tried, the more images of Bernie swirled through her brain. Maybe a drink. It wasn't part of the diet, but she could handle liquor.

She found a bottle of Amaretto in the kitchen cupboard. The taste of almonds filled her mouth and slid down her throat. She closed her eyes. Sweet Jesus. The warm syrup was a balm to the hollow within her. She poured a second glass. As she sipped the liqueur, warmth rose through her mouth to the top of her head. God, it was like an almond cake. This was childish joy: she was giving herself a birthday party. The almonds with sugar and flour and eggs could fill her body. She hated to leave the bottle. She wanted instant satisfaction. But it would take only a few moments to make a dough to taste like cake. She dashed about the kitchen gathering the ingredients. It would be hard to find everything she needed, for she had tried to empty the house of all foods not acceptable on her diet. She even avoided walking by sections in the grocery store where her favorite foods were kept. But there was sugar for Bernie's coffee; flour, a bit of flour for his gravies. She sucked on her finger as she looked into the almost empty canister. Powdered milk would stretch it. The Amaretto would cover any deficiencies.

The electric mixer growled as it chased the stick of cold margarine about the bowl. The blades nipped yellow slivers from the stick. She poured sugar into the swirling beaters. Grainy butter beaded the bowl. She cracked an egg. It slid into the mixture. For a moment the yolk stared up at her from its mucous pool like an accusing eye; then it whirlpooled into a cream. She wanted to stick her finger into the bowl, but the ferocious mixer stopped her. She dumped flour into the creamed mixture, and a mist of flour rose from the clogged beaters. The final touch was pouring about a jiggerful of Amaretto into the bowl to heighten the flavor. Every sense electrified for the climax, she dug her fingers into the mixture and licked them. As she gulped dough, her frenzy reached orgasmic culmination.

Her body felt stuffed to a level beneath her breasts when she looked up to see Bernie standing in the kitchen doorway. His presence was like ice water thrown in her face. His mouth opened slightly, his skin paled as he stared at her. "Thel?" He walked toward her. She felt as if she were thirteen and had been caught masturbating by her father. She grabbed a kitchen towel from the counter beside her and threw it over the dough, then blocked his view of the bowl with her body. He came to the counter, reached past her and picked up the bowl. She covered her face with her hands. "Thel." She slid her hands down her face so that she was peering at him from above the tepee of her fingers. "You eat this, Thel?" He stuck a finger in the bowl and licked it. He wrinkled his nose and wiped the mixture from his tongue.

She yanked the towel from the counter and began beating him about the shoulders and neck, shrieking. "You smoke and you drink and you sleep all the time." Then she began to cry, because nothing he did could compare with her strange, sick obsession. It was so disgusting. She was so disgusting. She hugged herself and turned her back to him. She wanted to die, to disappear. "I'm ashamed. So ashamed."

"Ah, Thel." He pulled her to him and rocked her.

She tried to push his arms aside, but she was weak with exhaustion. "I know I'm weird and sick and strange."

"Come on, Thel, I want you to tell me about it." He walked her to the living room as she dabbed at her eyes.

For ten minutes Thelma cried. At first she sat on the edge of the couch, rocking her head toward her knees and moaning. Bernie stroked her back, repeating, "It's okay." When she glanced furtively at his face, he caught her chin in his palm. His muddy brown eyes looked straight into hers, and he said, "It's okay." Then she let him pull her into his arms. It was a dream: the girl, the dough, this. It couldn't be happening to her.

Thelma drew away from Bernie and mopped her nose. "How can you say it's okay? It's weird, and it's sick, and it's awful."

"Everybody's a little kinky, Thelma."

She shook her head in disbelief at the absurdity of his remark. Could he accept this? She'd never felt so ashamed in all her life. How strange she must have seemed. She tried to see herself as he had seen her. She had always felt invisible when she binged. If no one saw her, then she didn't do it. But now—now he knew. She picked at her gummy fingers. "I'm trying to change. I'm going for help."

"Yeah?" His eyes were compassionate.

"I go to an organization." She didn't know how to explain O.A. It seemed so corny. He'd hate it. The talk about God. The really grotesque fat people. It was like bingeing. She pretended it was somebody else, not the real Thelma who went to those meetings. She liked to assume she wasn't as bad as "they" were; but she was, she must be, eating dough. Bernie was watching her closely, as if she had a rare disease.

"I've learned a lot. I mean, there are reasons why." She watched his downcast face. Reasons—how could she explain those reasons? He was the reason. He hurt her, he used her, yet she couldn't, wouldn't let him go. She couldn't even tell him what he did to her. She might lose him if she told him; then what would she be?

"It's okay, Thelma. It's really okay." He patted the back of her dirty hand.

"No, I really ought to tell you, Bernie; I really want to talk." She searched his face. He didn't want to talk anymore. It disgusted him too much. He would simply forget and they would go on. She would eat when she hurt and shut up and limp along until it was time to repeat the cycle again. No, Thelma, don't let it happen. Her words came in a rush. "I—we—don't talk."

He looked at her with surprise and hurt. He thumped his chest. "Talk? We're talking right now. We talk."

Her eyes were awash with tears. She looked forlornly at the wall. "See, Bernie, you don't listen." What was the use? It was hopeless. But maybe not. She should try to explain her feelings. Surely, now, he'd listen. "I'm telling you how I feel. That I feel as if we don't talk, and you tell me the way I feel is silly." She sensed that he was adrift in her strange rush of words, but she babbled on. "But can't you see how what I feel bothers me, whether it's true or not?"

"Yeah—well, yeah. I can see you're feeling very bad." He looked hurt. "So you overeat because you think we don't talk?"

"No, I—" She looked at her hands. It sounded so stupid when he explained it. It probably really was stupid. Did she want more than she could have? Those other married couples who looked so happy and chatty might really feel as separate and alone as she and Bernie. Maybe life was awful for everyone. She ate because she was lonely. She ate because she was tired. She ate because she couldn't stand not to eat. Because she couldn't stand to feel. "I—that's one of the reasons."

"So, I guess I'm a big problem for you."

She massaged her forehead. Dear God, he didn't understand what she meant. She herself wasn't sure what she meant. "I'm not saying it's your fault." She didn't know how she could make it clearer. "It's, it's the way I feel. I feel as if you just don't care about me. Because you don't talk to me. You don't tell me you love me, or touch me, except when we're in bed. And that—that girl tonight." She began to sob. How could she say it? She could not grovel. If someone didn't love you, if someone wanted to be with another person, you couldn't beg for his attention.

"Jesus, Thelma, you know I was drunk tonight. And, ah, I'm sorry about what happened. I really feel shitty about it. I never planned to do it. I just got drunk and she was there, and it just sort of snowballed."

She sniffed. "But why couldn't you spend time dancing with me when you got drunk? Why do you pick out some beautiful stranger?"

He shook his head. Unable to meet her eyes, he looked at his beefy hand on her shoulder. "It's just, ah, well, I thought you wouldn't be interested, you—"

"Wouldn't be interested? How can you say—"

He glanced at her face, then back at his hands. "Thelma, how long has it been since we had sex?"

She winced at his question and its blunt phrasing. "Made love? Well, I—" she tried to recall evidence to justify herself, but he was right. She'd gone to bed early, or gone to bed late, or said she was tired or had a headache. It had been so long, she was afraid to think of it. To make overtures was beyond her. What if he'd reject her? "Well, you never asked."

"Never asked? Jesus, Thelma. You're never home,

and when you're here, you're on the fuckin' phone or so goddamned nervous I'm afraid if I touch you, you'll fly into a million pieces."

She laughed—"Oh, Bern"—but he was right. Dieting had changed her disposition from its usual lethargy. She was restless and energetic; her nerves were raw. And she had to make her phone calls as part of the program. She made at least three a day, and sometimes people called her.

His face was victorious. "Well, it's the truth; you know it's the truth." He began to run with the line now that he had an opening. "You're always playing tennis or grading papers or on the fuckin' phone."

"Bernie." She caught his hand. A feeling of tenderness engulfed her. He was hurt. He genuinely felt neglected. His feelings had never occurred to her: she was embarrassed by her insensitivity.

He looked into her eyes. "Thel, I been wondering if you were running around. You're getting skinny, you're never home, you never sleep with me. Jesus, you're—"

"Oh, Bernie, that's so funny." It was hysterical: the thought of her having an affair. Who would be interested? She could never go through with it. They had been married for nine years, and she still undressed in the bathroom, or clutched her clothes about her as she changed so he never saw her standing naked.

"What the hell's funny about it? You're good-looking, an intelligent woman, and nice to be with. Dynamite in bed—whenever I can get you there, which ain't been too damned often."

"Oh, Bernie." She held his hand to her cheek. He seemed so vulnerable. "Dynamite in bed." How sad. How touching. She knew his sincerity by the intensity in his eyes. "Dynamite in bed." She had been so shy and frightened in the first years of their marriage that she hadn't had orgasms. His patience and gentleness had brought her out of her self-consciousness, let her join his passion, but they never talked about sex or spoke during the act. And when she became involved, she was amazed and somewhat shamed by their wordless lovemaking in the dark. Realizing that Bernie felt threatened by her, she almost started crying all over again. "Oh, Bernie, there are so many things I have to tell you."

"Yeah, I was afraid of that." He kissed her knuckles.

"Oh, it's not that at all. Not at all. You see, this organization takes a lot of time; there are meetings and phone calls and—"

"You mean it's a club you're messing with?"

"A club." She smiled as his face relaxed. Then she sighed and rested her hand on his shoulder. They looked into each other's eyes. Neither looked away. It was an embrace. Then they talked to each other and listened to each other for over an hour. Thelma felt as if she'd found a girlfriend. He was watching, he was listening, he was talking: he cared.

Bernie hugged Thelma and rocked her. "Oh, Thelma, Thelma. From now on I'm going to talk to you and you're going to talk to me and—"

"Let's try." She felt as if a dozen knots within her had loosened and unwound themselves.

He held her at arm's length and looked toward the opening in the drapes at the morning light. "Hey, Thel, for a couple of people who don't talk, we're doing okay. We've talked the night away. Want to go out for breakfast?"

She laughed. "Wow. Do you know what, Bern? It's the neatest feeling. I'm not hungry at all."

II.

Thelma wanted to give herself a gift to celebrate her tenth week of abstinence required by O.A. Ten weeks, and there had been only one slip from the food plan. Slip. A perfect example of understatement. Too bad the example was too weird to use for her kids in the classroom. Her departure from the diet had not been a slip; it had been a dive. She had plunged into eating with the despair of a suicide diving off the Golden Gate. She had tried to crush the image of Bernie's stunned face when he witnessed her dough binge. She wanted to shove it to a part of her mind where she would never see it again, but it was an indelible impression. It became the whip to keep her in line. Someone had seen her binge, so it had to be true that she did these strange things. Now she lived the O.A. program like a ritual: the diet, the meetings, the phone calls, the literature. And she was afraid. She dreamed of eating icing. Bingeing had given her some of the most ecstatic escapes she'd ever known. She must not ever let herself think of gorging. It was sick, bad, stupid, ugly. So each of her meals became an amulet to add to the string of the necklace wound around her neck to exorcise the demon who promised a moment of happiness in exchange for her self-respect. She must break the spell.

There must be a gift she could give herself to nurture her, to stop the nagging sense of denial which controlled eating made her feel. She tried to think of nice things other people did for themselves besides eat. Eating was the double-edged gift which she gave herself—a few moments of high, and a downer for the other ninety-nine percent of the time. A binge was self-inflicted suffering. She'd give herself the kind of gift healthy women gave themselves. Clothes. Women always gave themselves clothes. Shopping was supposed to be a delight. The thought of it terrified her.

She had exercised faithfully at the club health room and with her tennis drills. And she had fearfully weighed

herself once each month. The first month she had lost
fourteen pounds. The second she lost ten. They told her
to weigh only once a month. She didn't want to break a
single rule. In two weeks she could weigh again. The
baggy clothes which she had always worn to hide her
body hung on her now. She didn't want to shed her
cocoon. She would have to shop soon, but it would be
no pleasure to face the three-way mirror, to see her
dimpled flesh winking disgustingly from three different
angles. No, clothes wouldn't do it.

Hair. Women were supposed to like to get their hair
done. She could have something done to her hair. It had
been, well, probably fifteen years since she'd made any
major changes. In the teachers' lounge, Thelma asked a
young woman with a cap of hair wrapped around her
head like a raven's wing where she had gotten it cut.
The girl leaned forward and confided, "Mr. Edward works
miracles. Just put yourself in his hands."

Mr. Edward didn't bother with punctuality. Customers
waited thirty to forty-five minutes for his services. Thelma
had not seen him yet, and she had skimmed through
Vogue, Mademoiselle, and *Seventeen,* but she could
hear his voice and his patrons' giggles, floating from the
room where he worked his miracles. She wished she
had brought a picture of what she wanted. She wished
she knew what she wanted. To be pretty. To be trans-
formed. Flipping through the magazines, she saw a couple of attractive-looking photos, but she hated to tear up
his magazines or to carry them with her into his room.
She should just relax. She looked at the ashtray and
chewed at a fingernail, pulled her hand from her mouth
and glanced at it, then held it by its wrist in her lap. Ten
minutes later, a woman whisked out of the room. She
preened in front of the mirror, turning her head to ob-

serve both sides of the close-cropped cap that was identical to the one worn by the girl at school.

Thelma decided Mr. Edward probably weighed one hundred and twenty-five. He had the narrowest hips and wore the tightest pants she'd ever seen. She was glad she had on her smock top and dark pants, so she wouldn't have to view her circumference contrasted with his in the mirror. He was sweeping the last bits of the previous patron's hair into a long-handled dustpan, and he said "Hi-yah," as she seated herself in the barber's chair with a whoosh. He didn't seem to be looking at the total Thelma as he wound tissue around her neck, swirled a cape over her body and snapped the collar closed about her throat. "What can we do for you today?"

He pumped the chair so that she rose a few feet. She tried to turn to look at him, but she realized he wanted to converse with her face in the mirror as their focal point. She spoke to his reflection. "Well, ah, I'd like to change my hair."

"Umhum, umhum." He stared down into the nest of steel-gray and rust-colored hair and gingerly touched a few strands. "Badly abused." He swiped his fingers across her cape as if he were removing soil. Thelma wondered if it was an unconscious gesture or calculated to make her feel even more ridiculous than she already felt. He raised his black brows. "I'd say, gross neglect." He looked in the mirror to check Thelma's response and smiled at her look of chagrin. He clucked his tongue and shook his head as he scolded, "Naughty, naughty."

Thelma smiled. He was clearly a kidder. One of those strange, effeminate boys who learn to clown to survive. Probably dropped out of high school. Probably made twice what she did. Yet she was paying him and smiling, even though he made her feel as if her hair were a sour dish mop.

He was backing away from her chair. His close-set dark eyes almost looked crossed as he stared intently at her head. He clapped his hands. "I've got it!"

Thelma wished she could lift her hands from under the cape. It was too late to escape, and it was obviously useless to ask what he had in store for her. She said to the mirror, "I, ah, I liked the lady's hair who just came out of here."

Edward was collecting bottles from the cupboards. "Oh, no, no, no. Not the geometric look." He was putting on rubber gloves. "It is très chic, but—" He placed his rubber gloves on either side of her face and lifted the hair aside. They both looked grimly at her reflection. Same old silly-putty face she had given up on twenty-two years ago. The nose was too wide, the eyes too small, the forehead too narrow for the cheeks. The mouth was a stale frosting rose. "It would be too severe." He let her hair fall back into place like a spaniel's ears. "What you need," he was speaking to his reflection in the mirror, "is something soft, and light and high. You're a little pear-y, my dear. Your face, your body. We want to soften them."

Thelma shut her eyes. Peary. Of course he was right. How these faggy little boys must hate ugly women. And ugly as Thelma felt, she still felt feminine. She decided not to fight him. He probably knew his business. Some women looked beautiful in those stark haircuts because they'd look beautiful bald. When she opened her eyes, she'd commit herself totally to his mercy. Let him do whatever he thought he could do with the mess. He'd probably love the challenge.

The shampoo and conditioner, bleaching, coloring, curly perm, drying and comb-out took four hours. Once he began her transformation, Mr. Edward did not speak. Thelma was grateful for his honest lack of interest. It was a relief not to have to explain that she taught high school

English, not to have to listen to the usual responses: "Oh, I always hated English," or "Gee, I'll have to watch my grammar." Mr. Edward directed the girls to perform most of the mechanical, technical steps. They sopped her with lotions that burned her scalp or made her eyes water or smelled like sulfur. They banged the back of her head on the shampoo sink, or shoved her in and out of the dryer, where she burned her ears and the side of her face. Mr. Edward's specialties were styling and color. He whistled softly through his teeth as he leaned over her. She could feel his breath warm on her cheek. He was really sort of cute, with the skin on his high cheekbones shining and sparks in his brown eyes. As he danced about her performing the comb-out with a number of flourishes, he exuded an aura of cloves. She closed her eyes when he raked at her hair with a brush. She let herself go limp as he poked and prodded her. She was almost asleep when a mist of hair spray woke her. The hair in the mirror was no longer the color of rusting nails. It was blond with an apricot hue. It was a giant chrysanthemum of curls which haloed her head. The soft froth of hair turned her skin pinker and softer, and her face was no longer a pear. It was an egg. She smiled at herself. Even her wrinkles were muted by her hair. This was better. She turned her head to the right, to the left.

Mr. Edward handed her a mirror to view this minor miracle. "Better, huh?" He fluffed the top of her hair. "Low maintenance, too. Just shampoo and fluff dry."

"Really?" Thelma touched the back of her head. The hair was strangely soft.

"Well, you're obviously a low-maintenance type." He tilted her face back by the chin to give her one last appraisal. "The hair's good, but you really owe it to yourself to do something with your eyes." He let go of her chin, looked away and sniffed. "They're one of your best features, and they are totally lost with no makeup, which makes the top of your face look narrower than it really is. Emphasize those peepers. Especially with this. This blond stuff." He tweaked a ringlet.

An hour later, with three tones of foundation, blusher, eye shadow and freshly tweezed brows, Thelma paid in cash at the counter. The bill was twice what she'd estimated, but she had bought mascara, eye liner, eye shadow and remover cream, and a new foundation. If she didn't get the right kind, she wouldn't know how to do her own makeup.

Driving home, she was honked at twice at two different intersections. She wasn't aware that the light had changed. She was checking her hair and her face in the rearview mirror.

By six o'clock, when Bernie got home, she had begun to accept the woman in the mirror as herself. It had been a shocker. The hair was a little like Harpo Marx's, about that shape, about that color. But her face was a new color, and her eyes looked bigger. She looked a little like a handsome young man in drag. Fantastic what they did to themselves, those female impersonators. She looked— not pretty, but handsome, and better—much better—than rusty nails and faded eyes.

She waited in the kitchen for Bernie to walk in. He stopped in his tracks when he saw her and said, "Wow," three times. He laughed. He touched her hair as if it were cotton candy. Thelma expected him to lick his fingers. Then he looked closely at the makeup and said, "Wow," again and laughed.

Thelma looked at his eyes that looked at her hair and she asked, "Do you like it?" She tapped the shelf of his belly. "Bern, do you like it?"

He tilted his head. "Yeah, yeah. It's different. Rea

different. You look good. Yeah, you look great." He looked amazed.

She felt good all evening long. She didn't feel resentful eating her dinner of green beans, broiled fish and salad. She didn't begrudge Bernie his high-caloric additions of bread and butter, baked potato and chocolate cake. She decided that she had chosen a good gift for herself.

The next day at school she was a star. When she went to check her mail, the secretary did a double take. First-period sophomores whistled and stomped when she entered the room. Every class noticed. Even in the halls, kids whom she had never taught stopped her and asked, "What did you do to yourself?" The raven-haired girl in the teachers' lounge was impressed. Mr. Edward was a miracle worker, all right. But Thelma began to wonder—if they thought she looked so good now, what had they thought before?

That night Bernie came home early, and he bought a present. It wasn't her birthday or an anniversary, and he brought her a present. Carefully easing the ribbon from the package so that she could use it again, she wondered what was inside. She felt foolish and frightened. Something that she had always wanted to happen to her was happening. Bern had given her a gift as a complete surprise. She had not had to make a list as she did for Christmas or hint for weeks about her birthday coming. This was an unsolicited gift. Did her hair make so much difference? She was confused. She lifted the lid on the box. It was a tennis dress. An expensive brand. A sexy neckline. He had forgotten to have the tags removed. The flow of pleasure stopped. It was a size 10. She excused herself and went to the bathroom to try it on. Better to learn in private that the zipper wouldn't close around her sausage of a torso than to illustrate it before his eyes. But the zipper slid comfortably closed, the neckline dove provocatively into the swell of her breasts, and the skirt covered a number of imperfections. She looked almost pretty. Size 10. She hadn't worn that size since she was about that age. Of course it was an expensive dress. They always ran a little larger. But still. Giggling with pleasure and anticipation, she went to the living room to model the dress for Bernie.

—Rita Garitano

The Real Difference Between the Fatties and the Thinnies

At Last It Can Be Told ...

Every women's magazine has at least one such article and several ads. "Eat and grow slim!" one ad promises. "The diet for diet dropouts," proclaims the headline on the cover.

I read every one. I even follow their suggestions. For a whole day. Sometimes a week, a month, even a year.

But eventually, inevitably, I revert back to my old habits, letting the pounds slip back on, padding my ample hips.

But at last I've found The Answer. After living for almost fourteen years with a man who never gains an ounce no matter what I serve him for dinner, I've found out what it is that keeps him thin.

You see, I'm a Fatty and my husband is a Thinny. The

difference is not in our girth, our metabolism, or anything else that can be scientifically measured.

The real difference between the Fatties and the Thinnies is that Thinnies:

avoid eating popcorn in the movies because it gets their hands greasy.

save half a box of Good 'n' Plenty for later.

split a large combination pizza with three friends.

think Oreo cookies are for kids.

nibble cashews one at a time.

feed the leftover picnic sandwiches to the ducks.

complain that even one doughnut remains for hours an indigestible lump in their stomachs.

think lollipops are for kids.

read books they have to hold with both hands.

become so absorbed in a weekend project they forget to have lunch.

fill the candy dish on their desk with paper clips.

think candy canes are for kids.

counteract the midafternoon slump with a nap instead of a cinnamon Danish.

exchange the deep-fryer they received for Christmas for a clock-radio.

lose their appetites when they're depressed.

think chocolate Easter bunnies are for kids.

prefer *The Joy of Sex* to *The Joy of Cooking*.

save leftovers that are too skimpy to use for another meal in order to make interesting soups.

throw out stale potato chips.

think Cracker Jacks are for kids.

will eat only Swiss or Dutch chocolate, which cannot be found except in a special store.

think it's too much trouble to stop at a special store just to buy chocolate.

pass up the hot buttered rolls for melba toast.

think candy apples are for kids.

don't celebrate with a hot fudge sundae every time they lose a pound.

warm up after skiing with black coffee, instead of hot chocolate and whipped cream.

try all the salads at the buffet, leaving room for only one dessert.

think Rice Krispies marshmallow treats are for kids.

find iced tea more refreshing than an ice cream soda.

order a rare steak instead of roast pork with gravy.

get into such interesting conversations at cocktail parties that they never quite work their way over to the hors d'oeuvre table.

think peppermint patties are for kids.

have no compulsion to keep the candy dish symmetrical by reducing the jelly beans to an equal number of each color.

think that topping brownies with ice cream makes too rich a dessert.

bring four cookies into the TV room, instead of the box.

think banana splits are for kids.

—Barbara Florio Graham

My Mother's Prayer

"Eat and be thin.
Eat and be thin.
Eat, my child,
eat and be thin.

"Eat," she said,
"to make me happy.
 Eat," she said.
"I cook for you.
 I set your table,
 I shop for food.
 Eat, my child,
 eat and be thin.

"But don't eat too much,
 for if you do,
 you will be fat,
 you will be ugly.
 You will be fat,
 you will be lonely.
 No one will love you
 if you are fat.
 No one will *have* you
 if you are fat.
 Eat, my child,
 eat and be thin.

"Thin is good.
 Thin is beautiful.
 Thin is right.
 Fat is blight.
 Fat is ugly.
 Fat is lonely.
 Fat is bad.
 Fat is sad.
 Eat, my child,
 eat and be thin."

—Linda Myer

"If Only I Had . . .
Then I Would Be Happy"

The Body

I stared at Emily Patrino in the junior high cafeteria as she unwrapped her lunch: chocolate milk, Fritos, a tuna sandwich, an apple, and eight Oreo cookies. The cookies alone would have been, and often were, my ration for a whole day. Emily was a nice kid, but I couldn't stand her. She had skinny arms and legs. I wanted her body. I wanted to *be* Emily Patrino. Never mind about the rumors that she had a big mole on her left breast, that her father was a member of the Mafia, or that her mother walked around their house naked. She was thin, and that was enough.

Thin girls—and, later, thin women—enchanted and mystified me. I watched them in parking lots, supermarkets, department stores. How they walked, dressed, laughed; what they bought; whom they talked with; and, when I was close enough, what they ate. Being thin was, to me, the pinnacle of any life, the point at which you could throw in your cards and never have to accomplish another thing. Fame, riches and beauty paled in comparison to being thin; without the body, the accessories meant nothing.

When I got thin, my clothes size changed, I chilled more easily, and men I didn't want wanted me. When I got thin, I still thought I was fat. Being thin didn't bring me a lover or work.

I waited to get thin to begin my life.

And when I got thin, I waited for my life to begin.

Without the accessories, the body meant nothing.

The Dress

I wanted it, the dress in Folklorico. Twice I tried it on; made a special trip to Palo Alto, fifty miles each way. At night I imagined myself floating gracefully into a room, all eyes on me, the textured fabric draping over my legs, kimono cuts splaying around my neck. "I'll look prettier," I thought. "Things will be better when I have the dress."

Each night for two weeks I thought about it and always came back to: "Such a lot to pay for a dress. It's not worth the price." But its purple lushness glided, like a chiffon sash, into my heart. Every time something went wrong, I thought about the dress. It called to me with a promise of happiness: "Something that you didn't know was wrong will be right when you get me, when you get me, when you get me." And so my willpower collapsed.

For the third time in a month, I made the trip to Palo Alto. I bought the dress and carried it to my car like a treasure, placed it carefully on the backseat and hummed my way home.

The first time I wore it to a party, a friend walked over to me and said, "Where did you get that dress? I've never seen it before; it must be old." Before I could answer, she said, "It doesn't look like you—it's so dark and somber. But you know, it would make great pillows." Men didn't flock to my side, clamoring for my attention. Women treated me as they always had; the dress didn't make them like me any better. Then people started going into the bedroom, removing their clothes and filing out to the hot tub.

Before long, I was the only one in the house. Wrapped in deep violet elegance, I sat in the middle of the living room, eating potato chips and onion dip, wanting someone to talk to. Within an hour I had joined my friends in the hot tub, leaving my gateway to happiness crumpled on the floor.

The Work

When I realized, at twenty-one, that I wasn't going to be in college for the rest of my life and that I had to find something to do, I became like a wildcat: scratching, stalking, roaming. I moved from New Orleans to Buffalo to Bombay to Miami to New York to Big Sur. I jumped from job to job, went from counselor to secretary to switchboard operator to maid to dishwasher to apprentice doctor to astrologer. Scratching, stalking, roaming.

At night I would cry, wake up in a cold sweat, see spirits walking off the walls. I was haunted by the need for satisfying work, by a yearning that demanded release. I saw myself at sixty, at seventy, haggard and bitter; I feared that I would die unused.

Men floated into my life; they floated out. I'd stay with them for a few months and then I would leave. I wanted a career, not a man. A career would make me happy, happy, happy.

Now I have work. Exhilarating work. Fulfilling work. I live in one place; haven't moved for five years. But the focus, like a spotlight, moves swiftly, silently, to what I don't have, to a yearning that demands release.

At night, it continues, the scratching, stalking, roaming.

The Man

A man walks into the room. He has sky-clear eyes and Polynesian hair, blue-black and silky. I am talking to a friend about her child and watching the man out of the corner of my eye. He walks to the bar, pours himself a drink. He turns and leans on the wood, looks blankly into the room. I see him seeing me. His eyes stop. I pretend I am involved in the conversation, am listening with interest to samples of Susie's increasing vocabulary: "She can say *app-pull* now; she's changing every day." I feel his eyes on me. The edges of conversation about Susie become loose, and my friend drifts to the next group. The man weaves his way toward me. Someone stops him midway and they talk. Time for me to think: Is he the one? The man from *Esquire?* Is he the missing piece that will make my life work? Will I be happy, will I finally be happy if I am with him, if I have this man?

Our beginning would be ecstatic, the way beginnings have a tendency to be. We would watch the shadows of my palm tree making lazy patterns on the wall; we would spend days in bed, getting up only for cheese and wine and crackers. We would get the crumbs on the sheets and later we would laugh when they stuck to our naked bodies. We would make love until the days rolled into each other and piled into weeks, our time molding to the shapes of our kisses. We would crawl inside each other's smiles, rest lightly behind each other's eyes. I would become so attuned to his movements that they would become my own. His name would be my mantra. . . .

Ah, finally he is finished talking. Patting his friend on the shoulder, he glides to where I stand breathless, waiting.

Our eyes lock in an embrace. Silence. "I recognize you from somewhere," he says throatily.

Mustering my smokiest smile (right side of the mouth turned up farther than the left), I whisper a lie: "I recognize you, too."

"I think I've seen you at Eliot Cowan's shop. Don't you get your hair cut there?" he asks.

Reality sets in. Eliot's shop? What is the man of my dreams doing in Eliot's shop? I push my visions of shadowy palms and love-making in the afternoons aside for a moment. "How do you know Eliot?" I ask. "Does he cut your hair, too?"

"No," he begins. "Well, I mean, yes, yes he does. I live with Eliot."

"Live with him? But Eliot is—is—"

The dream man nods his head and grins unabashedly. "Your

name's Geneen, isn't it? Eliot's been telling me about you. Aren't you writing a book about chocolate?"

I mutter something meaningless.

Someone should have told me that the man from *Esquire* is gay; I wouldn't have waited so long.

Epilogue

Outside the night is balmy. I walk past two ruffly cats on a porch. They remind me of hooked rugs curled into each other. They stare at me, yellow-eyed and unblinking. I stare back at them and smile. Honeysuckle. I smell honeysuckle and turn to find its source. It's on a fence low to the ground. Burying my head in the tangled vines, I see myself jumping rope when I was ten. Summer and the first time I smelled honeysuckle. My friend Lucy and I made necklaces from it and bit off the white-belled petals, sucking the smell into our throats. I keep walking. Soon the click, click, click of my shoes hitting the pavement becomes a chant; my body pulses in rhythm to the sound.

When I get home, I wash, undress, slip into my flannel nightgown and crawl into bed. Clean sheets. The moon is washing over my room, lighting up the African violets on my desk. Outside, the copper wind chimes tinkle, lulling me to sleep.

In the moment between wakefulness and dreams, a question occurs to me: Could it be that happiness comes in moments—yellow-eyed cats, childhood smells, the glisten of moonlight, the clink of chimes? Could it be that I am already happy, that I have been happy all these years without knowing it, but that happiness passes, rises and falls, goes away and comes back?

I wake up content, and work while the day passes from amber morning to pale lilac afternoon.

Breaking Free

"We want to change in order to love ourselves, but
we've got to love ourselves in order to change."

—*a Breaking Free workshop participant.*

Breaking Free

Not long ago I was having dinner with a would-be lover. Over fettucine with cream sauce, garlic bread and a candle, he said, "I've been talking to my therapist recently about how difficult it is for me to say things to people that might hurt them."

My initial reaction was: "So why say anything at all?" which was followed by the thought: "Here it comes—something that he thinks is going to hurt me." My mind raced through the possibilities: He doesn't like my mother, my apartment, my friends; he wonders why everything I own is purple; he thinks I chew too loudly, talk too much, should kill the spiders on my bathroom wall. I waited.

"Well—uh—well . . ." he began.

"What is it, Michael? Whatever it is, it would be better said by you than fantasized by me. Please tell me."

"Well," he began again, "well, I have a question to ask."

"Yes?" I was beginning to get more curious than anxious.

"Well, would you like me if you saw me with no clothes on and you didn't like my body?"

"Of course," I said instinctively.

My mind's eye beheld an array of the different bodies I'd been close to: slender bodies with hair and muscles; paunchy, hairless bodies with flabby protrusions; classically stunning bodies, classically unattractive ones. As my memory played them out before me, flabby or firm, I realized that what I remembered about a body was the person who occupied it and the connection between us rather than the tone of his latissimus dorsal.

Divorcing myself from these swirling images of flesh, I looked closely at Michael, who was obviously waiting for something more from me. "Okay," I said, "now, it seems, the question to ask is whether you'd like *me* if you didn't like *my* body."

He flinched, heaved a sigh, turned his head away from the spot where our noses were practically touching, and whispered, "No, I wouldn't." I stared at the side of his head. A pimple was growing in his ear.

"It's been on my mind for a while, Geneen," he said, "and I feel that we've been so honest with each other that I need to tell you this, too. Ever since I've known you, the one thing that has gotten in the way of my seeing us together is that I prefer women who are thinner than you."

At that point I broke into peals of laughter. Now it was Michael's turn to stare.

"What are you laughing at? I thought this was going to be very difficult for you to hear, what with your focus on compulsive eating, your work . . ."

"I can't help it, Michael. I think it's all very funny. You've told me you're falling in love with me, and now you say that if you saw me naked and didn't like what you saw, you wouldn't be attracted to me anymore. My first response is astonishment—you already know the basic shape of my body—and my second response is that this attitude of yours must cause you a lot of pain."

Was that me talking? Me—Thunder Thighs, Moon Face and Apple Cheeks? Was that me laughing and yet feeling sorry for a man who was as much as telling me he thought I was too fat?

A similar scene, five years before, had followed a different script. Henry, a new lover, and I were jogging along the path that runs beside Niagara Falls, I in a black bikini and he in white shorts. Very nonchalantly, as if he were whispering to the wind, he said, "Your thighs are too big. You need to lose some weight." Continuing to run, I hid my tears and anger and hurt. I believed him and said nothing. I believed that it was *my* problem that Henry didn't like my thighs, instead of *his* problem that he didn't. I couldn't see that the real trouble was that *I* didn't like my thighs, which made me a vulnerable target for anyone—my friends, my brother, my mother—who preferred Farrah Fawcett to Dolly Parton.

When I became anorectic, I used my slowly disappearing flesh as a club with which to beat Henry. I hated him for telling me I was too fat.

"Is that all you have to say?" Michael asked, bringing me back to the present.

"No," I said without anger. "If I could have, I certainly would not have chosen this particular form, given the bony ideal of our society. Mine would have been taller, leggier, skinnier-armed. But since I wasn't consulted in the matter, and since I walk around in these curves every day, sleep with them every night and wake up with them again, I've had to make peace with them. Consequently, I've come to think my body is quite lovely and womanly. If you don't like it, Michael, that's your problem."

With those words, all the little people in my body who have been mowed under for years by the oppressiveness of fat judgments stood up and applauded. At the encore, I bowed to them and giggled out loud.

Speechless, Michael picked up his fork and dove into the remaining fettucine, adding a few more inches to the roll of fat hanging over his brown corduroy pants.

Breaking free is about realizing that other people's opinions of, judgments of, and projections onto your body have little to do with your body; they have to do with these people, their preferences, their values.

Breaking free is about the acceptance of your body and then the appreciation of it as the encasement that's carried you around for all these years. Except for a few minor setbacks, it has probably done quite well in spite of the abuse you've given it. Breaking free is about understanding that your body responds to *your* will, rather than having one of its own; it is misleading and inappropriate to treat it as if it has betrayed you and to dislike it accordingly.

Breaking free does not necessarily mark the cessation of bingeing (even thin people binge), although that may and usually does accompany the process. It does mark the understanding of the necessity to observe yourself when you eat so that you can discover whether food is truly satisfying the hunger of the situation. Self-loathing during a binge precipitates further bingeing because it destroys the sensitivity and awareness that can make you capable of exploring more satisfying forms of nourishment. You don't stop bingeing because it's disgusting, because you're spineless, or because you know you will be fat for the rest of your life if you continue. But the need to binge *does* become irrelevant when you realize what you want and that you will not get it by eating.

A woman I've worked with tells this story about a binge:

"On the same day that my lover told me he was leaving for two months, the family doctor called to tell me my mother was in the hospital. The next morning I woke up with a very loud voice in my head screaming, 'Doughnuts. Doughnuts.' For about two hours I was successful in ignoring it. Then I ate everything in the house that wasn't nailed down, until I finally decided it was time to get some doughnuts. Once in the doughnut shop, I ordered a glazed cruller. One wasn't enough, so I heard myself ordering another. And then a third. As I watched the fourth placed in front of me, I thought, 'Oh my God. I'm about to eat my fourth doughnut. I wonder what's going on.' It took me this long—from waking up to the fourth doughnut—to calm myself down. I wasn't freaked out that I was eating so much; I just looked at myself in amazement at what I had consumed. Finally, sitting in Alice's Doughnut Place with a policeman on one side of me and a truck driver on the other, I realized how sad and frightened I was about my mother and my boyfriend. I started to cry. Everyone looked at me like I was a little weird, especially the policeman, so I paid for my doughnuts, leaving the fourth one on the plate, and drove home. I spent the next two hours crying and sleeping."

Breaking free implies a redefinition of compulsive eating. Rather than being self-destructive, you are, on the contrary, trying to get through to yourself, trying to take care of yourself by eating. If you recognize that your wanting to eat when you are not hungry is an indication of a different kind of hunger, you can move from being the victim of a desire to a position of power and choice. You *still* may decide to eat, but that decision will come from awareness—not ignorance—of your needs and of the options available to you.

Given the difficult situations out of which your compulsive eating evolved, you can applaud yourself for having discovered a way to tolerate them. You did the best you could; food was an available outlet for your otherwise inexpressible feelings, and so you used it.

But you are no longer the child who was abandoned by your mother, taunted by an uncle, left by a boyfriend or girlfriend. When you began eating compulsively, you didn't have the tools, the words, the knowledge to express your feelings. Now you do. You can talk, scream, fight back, walk out, say no. Chances are, however, that you are still defining yourself in the context of what you perceive as past "failures," and that your sense of identity has been created from them with pieces of guilt, low self-esteem, and self-hatred.

Compulsive eating *is* resolvable. It is only your persistence in carrying past "failures" into the present that causes you to believe that a problem, especially that of compulsive eating, must repeat itself. You need to see that your responses to situations can and do change, that you really are different from the person you were ten years ago, five years ago, or yesterday. You have the capacity to respond from what you know and want *now*, rather than from what you knew or wanted as a child, or even as an adult a few weeks ago. There is no need to keep recreating your past.

Breaking free is not a wrenching process. You don't have to give up anything you are not ready to give up. When you break free from compulsive eating, it is not because you have proved yourself wrong. Breaking free is not a negation; it is an affirmation. Rather than attacking or destroying your behavior patterns, you focus on the source of the conflicts being expressed through your eating. Rather than attempting to change your behavior, you change the context; you change the framework in which you hold it. Your attitude changes from condemning yourself to acknowledging yourself.

Breaking free is a natural process, an evolution, in which you proceed from one step to another with awareness. Nothing has to be forbidden if you remain aware, which translates to observing your actions without negative judgment or guilt. Awareness may prove to be more difficult than it sounds. Your first response to pain is probably to try to leave yourself rather than remain with the discomfort. It's not easy to be depressed or sad without wanting to knock yourself out. And even harder to accept that no one can take your pain away. Sometimes the pain has to do with nothing more or less than your being alive.

Awareness requires a different kind of strength than dieting does; there are no rules to follow. Awareness asks that you go through an experience; if you are sad, let yourself be sad. Go to the bottom of your unhappiness instead of trying to push the tip of it away. Let yourself absorb it and move through it. Stay with it for a while—fifteen minutes, a half hour—then do something else.

Awareness also asks that, if you use food to knock out the pain, you notice whether or not it is effective; that you notice if and for how long the pain disappears. *Without* making yourself feel wrong for doing it, try to decide whether the food fills the ache, whether it does what you want it to do. If you learn that

food is not relieving your suffering—if it is, in fact, creating
more of it—you can choose a more satisfying anodyne. Not that
anything will actually dissolve despair; sometimes your options
are reduced to ways you can nurture yourself while the sadness
has a chance to wash its way through you. Some ways of killing
pain are more satisfying than others. And by remaining sensitive to the effectiveness of the methods on which you rely, you
are in a position to choose the ones that work. Eventually,
certain behavior patterns will fall away, like leaves from a
tree—naturally, gracefully—*not* because you are attacking them
but because you have no use for them anymore.

Breaking free is not a war, not even a fight. You don't divide
yourself into "good" parts and "bad" parts; the very attention
that this division gives to self-defeating behaviors often acti-
vates the patterns it is attempting to destroy. There is no need
to struggle, only to remain sensitive to the motivation behind
your actions and then to the *actual effectiveness* of those actions.
Breaking free is about trusting and strengthening your ability to
choose health over illness, growth over stasis. Given the
opportunity, you really can—and will—distinguish between
what you intuitively feel is wholesome and what is not.

The essence of breaking free is the kindness with which you
treat yourself. Your intention, when you begin eating, was
certainly *not* to make yourself miserable. You ate to protect
and take care of yourself. When you become conscious of that
intention, you can begin to trust your natural instincts, your
intuitive wisdom. You can begin to give credence to those parts
of you that, like a tropism, turn toward the light and the
warmth that infuse you with positive energy.

You live the way you eat. Your belief in yourself and your
ability to make decisions that will enhance your well-being
extend to every level of your life. If you deprive yourself of
food, you probably deprive yourself of other things, too. If you
feel that you cannot be trusted with food, you probably mistrust
your judgments, opinions and feelings. In exploring your rela-

tionship to food and hunger, you are tapping the foundation on which your self-esteem is built; the benefits of the time you spend in such exploration will, like the hub of a wheel, radiate to each spoke of your life.

When you begin experiencing the joy of providing nourishment for yourself on a physical level, the confidence in your ability to make other satisfying choices will grow. That confidence will, in turn, affect your friendships, your home life, your time alone. No longer will thoughts of food—what you just ate, shouldn't have eaten, are going to eat—occupy so many hours of the day, form the center around which your other activities revolve.

Be honest with yourself. Unless you are absolutely willing to face the truth about food and you (this means becoming aware of how much you lie, sneak, and cheat around it), you can't move. It is like looking at a road map: unless you know exactly where you're starting from, you can't find the way to your destination.

You break free with kindness, awareness, and love. You break free from the myths you have created about yourself: that you are basically untrustworthy and out of control; that you must change in order to be loved; that you must treat yourself with harshness and force in order to reach a goal.

Just as a balloon lies crumpled and flat until your breath fills it out, so your ability to be trusted and nurturing lies folded and unheeded in a corner of you. By focusing your attention on your worthiness, you breathe life into it—you give it space to move, to talk, to shimmer.

Breaking free is not especially about being a certain size or feeling like a "normal" person around food, although these results are concomitant with the process. When you start eating out of physical hunger and stop eating when you're satisfied, you lose weight. Being thin is not a blessing God gave to some people and withheld from others. Being thin is not magic.

In the end, you break free from the illusion that your hunger has to do with food and that the answer to it is being thin. You begin answering the call of a hunger that has never before been satisfied. You begin realizing your potential as the irreplaceable human being that you are, instead of using food to postpone that recognition.

Self-Hate and Rejection

The first mocha-capuccino cookie was a treat, something sweet to help stave off the anxieties caused by pressure. I deserved a second of my favorite confections after so many late nights studying and so much work left to do. The third cookie was comfort for the tension. The fourth was self-pity; the fifth was sabotage.

The sixteenth cookie had the sickly taste of too much sweet. My mouth was numb to flavor; my senses were numb to feelings. My jaw hurt from chewing with the speed of panic, and my stomach hurt from strain. A roll of fat reminded me that those cookies would keep me hungry for affection and physically unappealing. I knew I couldn't keep those cookies down.

I made myself vomit, using the practiced muscles of my stomach. Why do I do this to myself? Why do I stuff myself with self-hatred and shame, knowing I can never in this way get rid of the ugly anger and paranoia I'm filling myself with? Why can't I control myself? I carefully cleaned the toilet for the fourth time that day. Why can't I rid myself of my obsession with food, I wondered as I ate something to soothe my torn throat and to remove the sour taste from my mouth. Why do I hate myself, I cried as I reached into the refrigerator and began eating compulsively again.

At school the syndrome is called scarf 'n' barf, although none of us will admit their problem to another student, and few will admit it even to themselves. My therapist calls the syndrome bulimarexia and says I am not alone. Half her female patients have bulimarexia, or its cousin, anorexia. As many as one in five would-be-happy college women spend time hanging over a toilet seat.

No one can neatly explain the problem, but it starts with overeating. For me, food has always served as emotional anaesthesia and gratification. I was a fat child; not obese, but fat enough not to be able to climb the ropes in gym class when everyone was watching. Fat enough not to feel accepted, not to like my body, and never to have boyfriends.

I started the losing and gaining games early; I knew the calorie counts of most foods by the age of twelve, and had dropped out of Weight Watchers three times by the age of sixteen. By then my self-worth was measured only on the scale, and I was unhappy. So I ate.

I lost fifteen pounds before my freshman year of college out of fear, and lost another twenty that year by confining myself to the cafeteria salad bar and learning—for the first time—the pleasures of noncompetitive physical activity.

When I traded my thick sweaters for running shorts in the spring, I was startled at how much attention I got. Suddenly all the guys who had always firmly wanted to be Just Friends were interested in Going Out (and Going All the Way). I was the same person, but it was clear my attractiveness and weight were on an inverse scale.

I suppose that should have been no big surprise; I had only to look around me to see that desirable women my age were slinky-slim. All the Farrah-mascara media maids who proclaim that we must look like them to be attractive are *bony*. Their lean bodies are like powerless mockeries of the male physique. The models look male-weak instead of female-strong. The stereotype of a woman my age (any age) is ornamental, objectified, and sexually submissive.

I had always thought my brains were more beautiful than my body. It made me angry to think my personal appeal came from painted powerlessness. My needs to be true to myself and to be attractive started fighting with each other inside. I ate and binged to reject the stereotype I learned to reject food to be slim. All my old eating habits resurfaced; food was my panacea for any concoction of anger, boredom, pressure, fear, or loneliness. And I could have my cake and not eat it too. Vomiting became an automatic response to eating. There was no stopping the cycle. Vomiting emptied my stomach while allowing me to feed my compulsion.

There is no feeling of self-disgust like that experienced by a bulimarexic. There is no sense of shame like being in a bathroom wondering if anyone noticed how many times the toilet flushed, or if anyone noticed the smell. There is no embarrassment like being confronted about the problem by someone you care about, someone you think will forever consider you as distasteful as puke itself. There is no paranoia like thinking everyone may know about your problem. There is no self-hatred like feeling so out of control, so guilty, so disgusting.

I haven't vomited in a long time now. That's partly thanks to my therapist, a woman who helped me see that there's a lot more to who I am than what I eat and how I look. And I've made a promise to myself—not a promise to diet to get a perfect figure to be attractive, but a promise to like myself. All of myself.

My body is part of me—not an attachment or a tool for attraction. I've learned how it moves, and how it feels when it is strong and healthy. I feel alive. I've got pudgy thighs and a squishy stomach and I love them. For the first time I'm not on a diet, and I've stopped feeling guilty about food. Something at my center tells me when I'm hungry, and tells me when I really crave something utterly fattening, and then I can usually stop at one or two mocha-capuccino cookies.

Like an alcoholic, I will always be a bulimarexic. I struggle against taking that bite that will leave me a morsel too full, and sometimes I lose control. But I've stopped letting myself be controlled by the external— whether food or outward perceptions of appearance— and I've learned to listen to my inner self and to like that self. I've freed myself forever.

—*Laura Fraser*

Emergence

I find it difficult to give it a name, this thing, this problem. I could call it food, and that would be partly correct, because it is about being obsessed with food and feeling terribly deprived and undernourished; of longing for food and believing I do not deserve to eat. I could say it is about being a woman, and certainly it is inextricable from being taught that as a woman I must be beautiful, small, dainty; and if I am not these, then I am ugly and unlovable. It is about being bound and constricted because I am not this feminine image, but it is also much, much more. It is, then, an emergence, because this struggle is about knowing myself from the inside out and finding I am essential.

It will help you to understand if I tell you about my family. Every Sunday my family would gather at our grandparents' farm for lunch. Grandmother would prepare large meals with the help of her two daughters, Rosemary, my mother, and Linda, her sister. They cooked luscious dinners Southern style: Molasses-cured ham, pork roast, fried chicken, mashed potatoes drowning in butter, creamy golden gravy, sliced tomatoes and onions, hot buttermilk biscuits, corn bread, lemon cake and fudge pie. I loved to spread corn bread on my plate and cover it with butter beans and pile fresh scallions over the top. I was in Southern heaven. The meal was cooked and served by the three women and eaten by the men and the children. The women did not sit down to dinner with us but stood in the back of the kitchen, talking, eating furtively, waiting on us. They ate from plates the size of cup saucers. They were gorgeous women; my grandmother and my mother had the same prematurely white hair, strong cheekbones, full red lips, blue-violet eyes edged in black lashes and brows. My aunt was perhaps more exotic looking, with rich espresso-colored hair, olive skin and lips so full they were extravagant; they were voluptuous. Her sensual beauty was accentuated by her large round breasts and lovely curved bottom. I thought she was the most beautiful woman I had ever seen.

After lunch the men left the kitchen to watch football, play catch, go fishing or take naps. Then it was our time. We would clear the table and wash the dishes, and when the long glass table top was cleaned we sat down and waited while my aunt rolled the RCA Victrola into the room. She was in charge of selecting the records, and usually she began the concert with "Portuguese Washer

Woman" or "Walk In the Black Forest" because they were strong piano pieces. We played the kitchen table like a grand piano, pounding our fingers on the glass top, singing, laughing and belting out renditions of our favorite solos.

When our fingers were numb we moved into reciting poetry. My mother ached and moaned with A. E. Housman; Linda was immersed in Eliot, and Grandma often repeated the Whitman lines of which she was so fond, "I sing myself, I celebrate myself." I was their pride when I memorized, in full, Kipling's "The Female of the Species." After every refrain "But the female of the species is more deadly than the male," they would howl, "Amen, amen, amen!"

Our sessions were always followed by "girl talk." It was not the usual sharing of recipes, advice on child rearing, or cute stories about husbands and kids. It was instead discussions about dieting, cosmetics, clothing and beauty. I was fascinated by these talks, learning about the mysteries of being a woman; of smelling, tasting, feeling like a woman.

On these Sundays I listened to a long progression of new diets, from the three Oreo cookies a day, protein only, carbohydrate only, grapefruit before every meal, to my aunt's spit-out plan, her alternative to swallowing excess calories. I assumed this was the way every woman lived and ate. The alternative, they assured me, was mounds of flesh on their bones. I never saw any of these women overweight, ever.

There were several doctors in my family, one of whom staggered into the profitable sideline of helping women lose weight. He began giving my mother and Linda shots containing the urine of pregnant cows. This would, he said, speed up their metabolism, and they would lose weight rapidly. He cautioned them not to exceed five hundred calories a day and to eat no sweets, not even a stick of gum. The gum, he said, would set up a craving for sugar. To maintain their weight they had to stay on a low-calorie diet during the week, but on the weekends they could eat anything and everything they wanted. Many weekend nights my mother called to me from the kitchen, pleading with me to come help her stop eating. She would yell, "I am devouring everything in sight!" I thought then that she was kidding.

Her sister, my aunt, grew more anxious about maintaining her appearance as time went by. She took me on her rounds of drugstores, sending me in to pick up prescriptions from suspicious druggists for diet pills, laxatives and enemas. I was only nine or ten, but I understood her despair, her shame, and especially her sense of need. She bought thousands of dollars' worth of clothing and cosmetics until her parents were forced to close out charge accounts and tear up credit cards. She became too thin, losing her luscious breasts and hips, by alternately starving and gorging herself, vomiting anything she ate for fear of becoming fat and therefore unwanted. In the height of her despair she lit cigarettes and burned holes in her skin to prove her ugliness.

I began to develop breasts and hips but stayed adolescent-thin; food was not a problem but a pleasure. I was determined to transcend the women in my family; I had paid close attention to their ongoing pain and frustration. I was on the edge of becoming a woman—independent, autonomous, powerful. I felt as though fresh, new blood were coursing in my veins.

Yet, the confused feelings that accompany burgeoning womanhood, and the conflict between my personal desires and my family's obsessions overwhelmed me. My vital feeling about being a woman contrasted sharply with what I saw in life: the thwarted desires, smothered potentials and constricted, empty lives of the women around me. I withdrew and dove into food. In three weeks' time I had gained twenty pounds. My debutante "coming out" ball followed close on the heels of my sudden "fleshing out." I grew too fat for my dress. I habitually bought grocery sacks full of food—Oreo cookies, Sara Lee brownies, Twinkies, Fritos—and stuffed them voraciously down my throat. I became panic stricken; I felt I was smothering. I read *Cosmopolitan,* diet guides, *Mademoiselle,* anything I could find that would tell me how to lose weight. I became determined to learn how to diet. I did learn, and learned so well that I then became terrified to stop. I dieted for two years straight; two years of shutting down my sensory awareness. I tried not to smell food, taste food or be tempted by its color, texture or consistency. I tried to kill my needing or wanting *anything.* I felt dead; but I was thin—very, very thin.

A doctor friend of mine introduced me to ipecac, a medicine dispensed to induce vomiting in children who have swallowed poison. It could purge me, body and mind, when I felt I had eaten too much. I thought it sounded drastic, but I had gone for three months eating nothing but protein: tons of cottage cheese, farmer cheese, chicken, overcooked meat patties, dry, unsalted eggs. . . . Emotionally I was cliff-hanging thin; I knew that one wrong move or one strong emotion would start me gorging again. It was only a matter of time until it happened. Finally I bought two dozen brownies. I supposed I tasted the first one; I don't recall. I stuffed one after another into my mouth, ravenously gulping, choking, sobbing, cramming in more. When I had eaten them all, I drove to the drugstore, bought some ipecac and drove back home. I measured out three teaspoons of the syrup and chased it with warm water; it sent shudders through my body. I gagged and fought to swallow. I turned on the bathtub faucet, hoping it would muffle my retching sounds. I lay down on the cool white tile floor and waited. Waited until my mouth began to salivate and my stomach contract wildly, until I vomited everything, vomited until yellow bile was all that was left and the medicine was satisfied. My stomach empty, I fell asleep in exhaustion. As horrible as this experience was, I repeated it many times. I had to.

I then learned to be an expert vomiter without ipecac. It was for me a matter of survival. I had found the answer; never again would I be deprived of the foods I loved, never go to bed hungry, never experience the headachy, anxious hunger I had lived with for years. I could go to parties, go out to dinner with friends. I could eat whatever and whenever I wanted, as long as I vomited. In my mind the alternative was being fat, and that was intolerable. Fat had to it a monstrous quality. I heard my mother's voice saying, "I saw Virginia today and she has gotten grotesquely fat," or, "Nancy has given herself over to king spaghetti; her skin looks like a piece of lasagna. She's got a horribly thick neck, thick ankles, thick pudgy fingers. . . ."

I stared at myself in the mirror; did I have any of the dreaded thickness? To be thick, pudgy, plump or fat was to be hideous; and implicit in this assessment was that it was the woman's fault. She had let herself go. Surrendered, lost control, given up, neglected her looks . . . failed.

So I vomited. I would cram as much food into my stomach as I could hold, drink some water, bend over, push on my abdomen, and all would go well. I could vomit while driving a car, reading a book, washing the dishes. It was a well-worn part of my life, my day and my body. I was very methodical in this whole routine. I had devised an order to the foods I ate. For optimum purgeability I started with foods that were easy to vomit and took long to digest, foods such as cereal, bread, noodles, potatoes, pizza and hamburgers. I ate sweets last because of their speed in rushing into my bloodstream. I could never stand to keep any form of sugar in my stomach for more than five minutes, and I made very sure to put something else in my stomach before I ate the sugar. I learned that certain foods such as doughnuts, chocolate, and peanut butter sank like bricks to the bottom of my stomach and had to be dynamited out. There were whole days I could do nothing but eat and vomit hour after hour until I fell asleep. On those days I was usually unable to leave my house, and if I did it was only to buy more groceries. My room was littered with brown grocery bags; my closet stuffed with empty cartons, boxes, and cans. On good days I could wait until night to binge and vomit; but when I became what I called "functional," I did not binge, but ate and vomited each meal individually, thus freeing my evenings for work, reading and friendships. I did not, during the seven years it lasted, think of easing up on myself. I did not even consider the possibility that what I was expecting of myself as a woman was wrong. I *did* think I was crazy or damaged; I felt that I could not expect to function normally. For me to sit down to a meal without fear and pain, eat the food and let it nourish my body, seemed inconceivably out of reach.

I do not mean to oversimplify, to suggest that it is all a matter of thinness, of body image, and of woman being objectified. It is a tangled problem. It also has to do with needing to feel in control of one's body, of mastery and accomplishment. It has to do with pent-up rage, sadness, power and strength—combined with one's ambivalence about being female. Women, I felt, did not deserve to eat. Women didn't work and produce like men, and they didn't use up energy like men, so they didn't earn their food. They ate like birds. I did not believe that I could be both beautiful and intelligent and still be loved. I learned that a woman's sole purpose was to be beautiful for others, and so there was no place for my need to be competent, powerful, expansive, wild and visible (all of which I was sure were strictly masculine qualities). I expressed all of these needs in vomiting. I could do what every woman I knew wished she could do; that is to eat everything I wanted, as much as I wanted, freely, and still be thin, petite and pleasing to others.

If this reads as if I am trying to justify what I did, I am. I can understand why any woman would express herself in the same way. I knew all the years I was vomiting that I was trying to survive and to expand the part of me that is strong and enduring. The price I had to pay became more than I could afford. I became severed from my body's natural responses and needs. I was always hungry and undernourished, and so I continuously craved and fantasized and wanted food. All food was "forbidden" to me, and so it caused anxiety, whether it was a salad or ice cream. There were a few foods like yogurt and fruit that were okay for me to eat, but even with those, if I felt too full, out they came.

When the pressure became too great and when I realized I could not change on my own, I found a therapist who told me I could trust myself. I began attending a women's support group dealing specifically with eating problems. There I learned that instead of using food and vomiting to do and say things for me, I could express them in my life. My emergence is slow; it's like untying knots in a fine silver chain, one at a time and with care. I was assured by these women that I could trust my body, my hungers, my needs and desires. I began in fantasy, imagining myself buying all the foods I wanted, taking them home and filling my cupboards and refrigerator. I felt secure in that fantasy, so I tried it in actuality. A little bit at a time I brought foods home, starting with fresh vegetables and salads with real salad dressing (you know, with mayonnaise and sour cream?), and then breads: thick homemade wheat breads, cinnamon and raisin breads, dark rye, bagels and corn breads. After a while I could even buy butter to spread on the bread, then peanut butter, followed by grape, raspberry and strawberry jams.

I chose one food per week, and with the help, nurturing and compassion of the women, I began to eat and to allow the food to stay in my stomach to nourish me. The first full meal I ate was at a potluck given by the support group. When the food didn't transform my body into a mountain of flesh, as I had believed anything fattening would, I began to trust my body again.

I have experienced bouts of rage at a society that would drive women to seek acceptance through fashionable emaciation, rage at what I was taught at home, and rage at myself for denying and distrusting who I am. I still have waves of grief for the woman I smothered and silenced for so long. My response to hunger and food is slowly becoming natural, easy, and pleasurable. I feel solid; I feel beautiful from the inside out. And I know now that beauty has nothing to do with looks; it must be felt.

I have a fantasy that I repeat to myself, instead of turning to food, when I need comfort and nurturing. I am at a celebration with hundreds of other women. It is a summer evening, about dusk, when fireflies begin to play. It is warm and the smell of honeysuckle is strong. We build a fire and set tables around it covered with lovely embroidered cloths. We bring out a glorious array of foods: roast chicken, turkey, potatoes, yams, large colorful salads, nuts, hot wheat breads, platters filled with fruit—pineapple, papaya, mangoes, apples, bananas, figs, dates—whipped cream, cakes and pies, wine and rich coffee. A feast for women, not one where the food is prepared for men to enjoy—or one of those horrible parties where the women gather guiltily around the food table and pick furtively. We eat and enjoy every bite. I add various pleasures, depending on my mood; sometimes we pile all the *Cosmopolitans, Vogues, Seventeens* and *Playboys* on the fire and sing as they crackle and spew. Always we dance and sing, and finally I lie back on the cool fragrant grass. The fire warms the night air. Staring at the stars, I know that this world is mine. I feel the food in my belly, feel it nourishing my body, feel the laughter and strength in my bones; and I am completely and overwhelmingly satisfied.

—*Rachel Lawrence*

The Way Out

December 30, 1980

Eight P.M.; kids asleep; the time I have been waiting for. I pour myself a glass of wine, butter a slice of bread, and climb into bed. This is my first glass of the day—I don't let myself drink before the kids are in bed. The glass empties fast. I get up for another and for more bread and butter. How many glasses do I drink? How much bread do I eat? After three or four glasses I lose track. Between 10 and 10:30 P.M. I lose consciousness.

I drink compulsively. I eat compulsively. I cannot stop myself.

During the Christmas season of 1980 I acknowledged how my body felt. Every morning I woke up with a thick, fuzzy grayness filling my head. It took hours to become fully awake. I knew I was gradually gaining more and more weight. The mirror told me that I was aging quickly. "If I keep drinking like this I will be dead in ten or fifteen years," I heard myself say out loud one night as I sat in bed drinking. "If I can hang on for fifteen years, the kids will be old enough to take care of themselves, and then there will be no reason to live. I don't have the courage to commit suicide, but the food and the alcohol are doing it bit by bit. I want to die. This is a way to do it."

My actions had finally found a voice.

January 4, 1981

I resolve to stop drinking. Now, today. I did it once before, for three months, and the physical stress alone was immense.

I have been on a million diets. I know the deprivation and the anger that I experience when I limit my food intake. To give up alcohol—the substance I use to give myself the ultimate secret treat—is going to be an experience far worse than any diet.

I am going to need help; I cannot do this alone. I will write in my journal every day. But the drinking and the eating have always been done in secret, and I know instinctively that I also have to find myself a public place for support. I think of Geneen's classes for compulsive eaters. I decide to ask Geneen if I can join her class. Not to lose weight, or to deal with my compulsion to eat, but as a support place to break this addiction to alcohol.

January 10, 1981

Geneen agrees to allow me to join the class as an alcoholic, but there will not be an opening for me for over two weeks.

January 18, 1981

The first two weeks of not drinking, of total withdrawal, were over today. I knew that it had to be cold turkey; I knew my body was going to be shaken to its roots. I had been drinking wine regularly for the last ten years, always a little more, a little more. Ten years—with breaks for pregnancy and lactation—is a long time. The times without alcohol were minimal in the whole picture. I needed to do those first two weeks alone. It was so tremendously difficult, I felt I had to be alone at the beginning. No questions; no one looking at me, wondering how I was doing, if I was going to make it.

Am I going to make it?

January 29, 1981

First meeting of Breaking Free. I am absolutely terrified. I know that Geneen will have us say something about why we are here. I know that I need to make a public statement. To say, "I am an alcoholic, I drink compulsively, I need to ask for support."

When I walk into Geneen's living room I am overwhelmed by a sea of totally unfamiliar faces.

The tension in the room is thick. One woman speaks to Geneen; the rest are very still. Soft music plays. I feel that I am going to shoot right through the roof, propelled by the fear that is pumping through my body and the bodies of all the other women.

The class starts. The door is all the way across the room from me. Why did I sit here? I can't get out unnoticed. I will not say a word, I tell myself. Even though I know it is important to say why I am here, I feel I cannot talk. These women only deal with compulsive eating; they are only overeaters. They are not compelled to eat *and* drink until oblivion sets in.

Geneen does the preliminary introductions. "Now ▶

would like each of you to say a little about why you are here," she directs.

I do not *have* to talk. I tell myself this over and over again.

The first one who speaks is a stalwart-looking woman with short brown hair. "My name is Rachel," she says. "I am a recovered alcoholic. I have been dry three years, but now I am overweight. When I first stopped drinking I lost twenty pounds; now I have gained them back and more. I hate my body. I hate this constant struggle. I just wish I could cut pieces of it off."

I cannot believe what she has said. She said the word alcoholic out loud. She said it to the whole group.

Other women spoke. "My name is Diane," said the curly-haired woman in the flowered blouse. "I lost sixty pounds at the Weight Place and I need to lose another sixty pounds. I can't seem to lose any more. They suggested that I try Geneen's class."

"My name is Maria," said a slimmish woman with long brown braids. "It's hard for me to talk about this. I can't really say very much tonight, but I need to be here."

As the words came out of the other women's mouths, I slowly gathered courage to speak.

"My name is Florinda. I stopped drinking twenty-two days ago. I have been drinking for ten years. I am here because Geneen said that I could use the group as a place to deal with my compulsion to drink. I am overweight; I know I eat too much. I have been overweight for years, but I don't want to lose weight. I just want help to try to stop drinking." I looked directly across the room into the face of the woman with the short brown hair. Rachel smiled back at me.

I think I may have the support group I so desperately need.

February 2, 1981

Dear Alcohol,
    I am giving you up to survive. But how can I nourish myself without the nourishment that I gave myself with you?

                              love,
                              me

    The guided fantasy that we did the first meeting at Geneen's stays in my mind. We went on an imaginary trip to the supermarket. All I wanted at the store was the touching of other people's bodies. I do not want food and wine as much as kisses and tongues in my mouth.
    There is a direct connection between my mouth and my pelvis. As though I take food and alcohol into my mouth to feed the aching hunger in that deepest part of me. I have kept it hidden away for years. Swallowing it with the alcohol and food. Trying to keep it down, way down.
    Now that I do not have alcohol to numb and blur, I am beginning to feel the hunger sharply and clearly. What do I do with this hunger? I have been celibate for four years now, since Michael and I separated.

February 5, 1981
    Second meeting; same women, same room, Geneen in the exact same place; and yet it all feels different. I want no one to notice me. I wear dark pants and a dark blue shirt. My hair is pulled back tightly. I do not say anything tonight. It's been a month and a day since I stopped drinking. I've binged on food for the last two nights, eating until my stomach cried in pain and still not wanting to stop.
    Maria talked tonight. She said she put empty boxes in

the cupboard. "I eat everything in the boxes, like crackers or cereal, and then I put the empty box back in the cupboard so that my husband will not know I have eaten it all. As soon as I can, I go to the store and replace the box. The problem is that we live in the mountains and it is not easy to get to the store. Sometimes it is three or four days before I can get there. I worry constantly that he will find one of the empties.

"Ice cream is the worst. I can eat a half gallon of ice cream at a time. He likes ice cream too. I live in terror that he will go to the refrigerator some night and find the empty carton and realize that I have eaten the whole thing."

"Do you ever eat like this in front of him?" Geneen asked.

"No, oh no! He'd think it was awful. He is never excessive. He is very careful about his body. He would never understand why I do this." Maria's face was very tight about her mouth.

"Do you think that maybe you leave those cartons in the cupboard so that he *will* find them?" Geneen asked gently.

"Why would I want that?" Maria's eyes were incredulous.

"Maybe there is something you are trying to say to him with all those empty cartons that you feel you cannot say yourself," Geneen told her.

I thought about the empty wine bottles that I used to keep in the refrigerator. Even when I lived alone with only the kids and no adult to find them, I put the empty bottles back into the refrigerator. Some nights I even filled them up with water so it looked as if I hadn't drunk at all that night. After the kids were in bed I would make secret trips to the store to buy more; I never seemed able to bring myself to buy wine in the daytime when I bought the groceries. It surprises me that Maria feels the same about eating crackers and ice cream as I do about drinking wine.

February 6, 1981

Drank to numb my desire for sex.

Tonight, here in bed, I made a list of all the men in my life whom I have been attracted to, wanted to make love with. I make a list of all the women I have been attracted to. The lists are much much longer than I expect.

For years I have swallowed my voice. I have tried to act out the roles of the good daughter, the virtuous wife, the kind mother. I married to console my mother for my loss of virtue. I wasn't strong enough to displease her and say, "No, I don't want to marry this man." I never let myself even think about any other man I might have been attracted to because a good wife loves only her husband. Then my kids were born and I swallowed even the sexual feeling that I had allowed for Michael. The sexual voice, that sensual core, was buried deeper and deeper.

I sank down. I disappeared. I gave myself alcohol and food. Instead of speaking my voice out, I took in.

I want to give myself a sense of myself. Hearing my own voice will eventually be what will enable me to leave behind the addiction to alcohol and food.

February 8, 1981

My parents are visiting. My mother cooks dinner. I feel panicky. They drink wine with their meal. Will I be able to get through without my familiar friend to protect me?

I make it, but at a cost. I feel fragile and shaken. I sit here in bed now, the house quiet, everyone in bed; and I realize that I have no memory of the taste of the food.

February 12, 1981

When I walk into Geneen's, I greet Rachel and sit next to her. The heavy woman with the flowered blouse and curly hair greets me politely, and Maria smiles as I sit between her and Rachel.

Once class starts we do a fantasy. Geneen tells us to imagine ourselves at a party as fat as we can possibly become. I see myself in a gray net dress, with ruffles and flounces all over it. It is immense, with a huge skirt. Then we imagine we are at the same party as slim as we have ever wanted to be. This time I see myself in a backless black gown. I am surrounded by people. I end up hiding behind some roses in the garden. I cannot get away.

When I am fat, people stay away from me. I can leave by mentally slipping out of my huge body. But thin, I am unable to leave the uncomfortable situation. I am out of control.

February 26, 1981

I am going to attend my first party since I have stopped drinking. I do not like parties, but it is my sister's birthday. Everyone will be drinking. How will I get through it?

Geneen suggests that I drink soda water. She suggests that I visualize what I will do at the party—how I will act. See myself feeling comfortable.

It is difficult to visualize. When I finally manage, I see myself being very quiet.

March 2, 1981

I went to the party. I drank plain soda water. I did fine.

March 5, 1981

Sixty days that I have not been drinking. I have lost five pounds. I wake up in the morning without a headache, feeling good.

March 12, 1981

Rachel and Diane save a place for me between them on the cushions.

"What happened to the woman who had the drinking problem?" Diane asks. "Remember her? She was here the first night."

"That was me," I say.

"You! But you aren't anything like her."

March 19, 1981

I sit next to Maria. Every week she has come to class looking fuller and fuller in the breasts; her face is changing subtly too. I wonder if she is pregnant.

Geneen turns off all the lights but one very dim one. She tells us to get up and close our eyes. I feel scared. She puts on music, tells us to move around the room with our eyes closed until we connect with someone. When we connect we are to stay with that person. Rachel and I bump into each other; we stay together.

Geneen tells us to touch each other, to feel each other's heads, faces, shoulders, arms, bodies, legs and feet with our eyes closed. I touch Rachel first. Starting with her head and face, I move down her torso to her thighs, calves and feet. I feel her bones, her strong neck, her chest and breasts, the strength in her back. I feel the soft roundness of her curves. She is luscious, strong and firm.

When it is my turn I feel myself tensing, trying to ward off the touch that I know is coming. She starts with my head. She moves slowly, tenderly touching breasts, back, hips, thighs. I begin to let go.

She moves down my legs to my calves, strokes them. Up and down she moves her hands, and I feel I am slipping into a dream. Michael's face drifts into my consciousness. Michael used to stroke my legs. How long has it been? But Michael's face is supplanted by my mother's face. My mother's face—and there are tears streaming down *my* face.

My mother. Oh Mama, Mama, I want you to stroke my legs. I have tried so hard to make you want to do this. You, Mama, before there was anyone else. I am little. I cannot talk, so small. I am in the dark. Mama's hands on my legs? I need her hands on my legs. Touching my legs, rubbing my legs. Mama, Mama!

I have slipped into my legs, into a part of me before words. It is dark; all is dark. I can hardly leave the exercise and come back into the room and the other women and the light. I leave the class stunned.

Now I am here in bed. I am filled with aching. This ache has been in me almost as long as I have been me. Aching for my mother's touch. Aching for my own touch. Aching to be in touch with me.

Alcohol numbed that ache. What do I do without you, alcohol? You were my lover for so long. You kept this ache at bay. Why did I let you go?

March 21, 1981

I have been thinking about what Rachel said after the touching exercise.

"There are parts of my body that I never let even my lover see. After three children and now that I am over-weight again, this part of me is flabby and ugly. It really bothered me to have it touched. My lover is younger than I am. I cannot bear for anyone to see how ugly this part is. I only make love in the dark. I turn that part away."

There are parts of all of us that we keep in the dark, do not let anyone see or touch.

April 2, 1981

Last night of this group with Geneen. Have not been here since we did the touching exercise. Too much coming too fast. Our dog Marco died, and then I drank that night. Thank goodness I have not drunk since then. On April 5 it will be three months I have not been drinking.

I have done some very good, hard work. This group has given me support on so many levels. Lots of changes—subtle changes. There is movement. The iceberg is defrosting.

Rachel and Diane are going to take the class again when it starts in May.

Maria announced that she is pregnant. The baby is due the end of July. "I am not sneaking food anymore. I eat what I want to eat right in front of my husband. It was pretty scary at first; now it feels just great." She smiles. "I even eat what I like to eat."

Rachel looks at me. "Are you going to take the class again?"

"I don't know. I have so little money. I just don't know."

"I sure hope you do," Rachel says.

April 16, 1981

In spite of the chaos of the past week—an old friend visiting with his kids and many upsets—I did not take a drink. I did not even overeat; how amazing.

April 26, 1981

My eating habits are changing. How is this happening? I am not eating bread and butter anymore. I just do not want it. It's been a whole week that I have not thought about taking a drink—a whole seven days without thinking about a glass of wine before I go to sleep.

I am aware that a lot of the time I eat food that I don't even like. I don't stop eating it, but at least I am aware.

April 30, 1981

Eleven A.M. I sit at the typewriter and write. The quiet of the house seeps into my bones and nurtures me.

Writing is a way of being alone with myself. I have been so lonely for myself for so long. I have missed myself at so many corners.

Writing nurtures me in a way that alcohol or food never has. I feel guilty taking this time in the middle of the day to write. I feel I should be eating leftovers or cooking—not writing in my journal in broad daylight.

May 4, 1981

Four months today since I stopped drinking. Michael, my ex-husband, got married today.

While the kids were away at the wedding, I spent the time washing the dishes. I washed slowly and steadily with the hot, hot water and great puffs of soapsuds. I took a long break in the middle to have a cup of coffee and eat a raisin bagel.

I did not overeat. I did not drink. I went to bed early.

May 7, 1981

Start of new Breaking Free class. It feels good to be here. I am excited. Rachel is not here, but will be next week. Maria is wearing a pregnant-lady smock—looking radiant.

I wonder why it is I want to be heavy? Heavy like a mother? To mother myself?

Goals for this class:

Learn how my largeness relates to how I see myself.

Find out what I really want to eat and where I want to eat it.

Discover what really nurtures me physically, spiritually, emotionally.

We do the fantasy of the fat lady at the party and the thin lady at the party.

The fantasy has changed a great deal. I am the big mother. I am tall, big-boned, heavy. I am alone in a high-ceilinged room. I stand awkwardly. The others are not in this room. There are two rooms off this large room. In one room there is dancing; in the other, food.

After a long, long time I finally let myself go into the room where the dancing is going on. I dance, large and fat and heavy.

I am thin. I am wearing a pretty white dress. I dance and dance and dance. I do not stop dancing.

Why don't I dance more?

May 14, 1981

How does play nourish me? How do sex and play fit together?

The original sex play with Michael was loaded. I was a virgin. I wanted sex; I wanted to play around, to just enjoy sex. Sex with Michael was the most joyous play I had ever known. It was as if someone had shown me a whole new playground. Then we got married. I didn't want to get married. I stopped playing. I gained twenty pounds the first year we were married.

Being fat keeps me safe from becoming involved again in sex play.

Being fat is my comfort, my hugs and kisses.

Being fat protects me from being seen by the world.

Being fat keeps people from seeing how vulnerable I am.

Fat keeps me looking grown up so that people don't know what a child I am.

The fat protects the child. The child stays untouchable and unhurt because I have entombed that part of myself in my fat.

May 16, 1981

I like to eat outside in the garden better than in the house. Why don't I have a table and chairs on the deck?

May 21, 1981

Rachel comes in radiant. She is wearing a soft pink blouse, a pink tee shirt, soft drawstring pants. Her skin and face glow. She looks as though she has lost twenty pounds.

"Rachel, have you lost weight?" Geneen asks her.

"No. Actually I have not lost a pound," Rachel says, beaming. "John, my lover, has been away teaching down South. Last weekend I went down to join him. We stayed in a motel. Do you know what?"

Everyone was listening; Rachel's voice was joyous: "I didn't wear a stitch of clothing the entire weekend. Well, that's not entirely true. I did dress when we went out to eat." We all laughed. "John kept telling me I was beautiful. How much he loved to make love with me in the daylight. We took showers together for the first time. We gave each other baths. I kept looking at myself in the mirror."

This is the woman who would only make love in the dark. This is the woman who wanted to cut the fat off her body.

Geneen asks us to make a list of the ways we keep ourselves deprived.

1. I do not play.
2. I do not tell people when they are hurting my feelings.
3. I do not allow myself to go out among people where I would meet and be with others in the fear that I will once again be hurt, stepped on, shunted aside, bounced on like an inner tube that has no feelings.
4. I keep myself deprived by not eating what feels nourishing to my body.
5. I do not allow myself to dance, play, laugh, talk.

May 22, 1981

Tonight I am not drinking, but I am eating: bran muffins, ice cream, washing them down with half-and-half. I want to coat and soothe my stomach with this food, but it still hurts. Why is my stomach in pain? Sometimes I think that I rush around blindly, hurrying, grabbing food and stuffing it into my mouth, unable to focus on details— because I am afraid if I focus I will feel all this pain.

May 25, 1981

The kids and I had dinner out in the backyard. I love watching the birds.

May 28, 1981

We make a list. I write—
I am waiting to get thin to:

have flowers in the house
wear soft fabrics, bright colors, clothes I like
swim in the ocean
make love, engage in sexual play
climb a tree
tell people I am little and they can easily hurt me
write my novel

June 1, 1981

I have hay fever badly these days. I notice also that coffee makes me nauseated, and yet I continue to drink it. It seems a bit like drinking alcohol. All those signs that alcohol did not work for me, and yet I kept drinking—still want to drink.

What is this compulsion not to listen to myself? Do I really enjoy coffee? Obviously my stomach doesn't. Where is the communication breakdown?

June 4, 1981

I did not go to class tonight. I feel too miserable. I can hardly breathe. I do not have the energy to confront myself tonight.

June 10, 1981

I see my acupuncturist. She tells me the hay fever and the tender, sore stomach are related. "No coffee," she declares first thing. "No milk, no beef, no sugar—no sweet stuff of any kind, not even honey. Can you do this?"

I hear myself say that I can do this.

June 11, 1981

"Tonight," Geneen says, "I want you to close your eyes and visualize the parent you have always wanted to have. It can be anyone you know or someone you've never met."

It is very difficult to do this. The vision of the guardian only comes in vaguely; she is fuzzy and indistinct.

"Now I want you to write down all the things you want this guardian to say to you."

The guardian tells me:

"I love you.
You are beautiful and wonderful.
I like you just the way you are.
There is no one else like you.
I am your friend and ally.
I like your body, your stomach, your buttocks, your legs and arms and breasts and feet. I like every part of you.
I like to watch you.
I like the way you walk.
I like the way you run.
It gives me pleasure just to be with you."

"Now," Geneen says, "find a partner." Rachel becomes mine. "Your partner is going to read your list to you. She is going to hold you or stroke you or whatever it is that you would want your guardian to do."

I feel the cold crunch of fear in my stomach. I find I can only breathe through my mouth. I would like to leave. I am to go first. Rachel strokes my calves; I ask her to. She reads my list to me. She reads it over and over again. I am crying. I am crying and crying and crying. It feels good. My God, does it feel good.

Then it is Rachel's turn. I stroke her forehead. I read her list to her. Her face is smooth, relaxed, soft and glowing. We hug for a long time when the exercise is completed.

June 18, 1981

It has been five months and fourteen days since I stopped drinking. Now I am not even drinking coffee. My stomach is feeling better. I weigh ten pounds less than I did when I started this group in January.

Diane has moved. "You know what," she told us, "in the stress of finding a place and moving, I didn't gain even a pound. For me that is just incredible. I mean, it's almost the same as losing twenty pounds would be for someone else."

We all clapped and clapped.

June 25, 1981

This is the last night of class. Geneen is not going to be teaching this workshop over the summer. I feel that it is time for me to stop, but I feel deeply saddened to leave all these fine brave women. These are the same women who were so alien that first night. It makes me smile with joy to think how far I have come in such a short time. Without the help of this group and Geneen I do not know if I would have been able to do what I set out to do. The work is not done, but the first and hardest part of it has been accomplished.

AFTERWORD
November 21, 1981

It has been ten months and seventeen days since I stopped drinking. I have, without dieting, lost ten more pounds over the summer, which makes a total of twenty pounds. People ask me now if I am losing weight. "Yes," I reply, "I seem to be doing that." My face looks younger to me, revealing an old beauty that I have not seen for a long, long time.

I consider myself a recovering alcoholic. Ten months is not really a very long time when compared with ten years. Each day I do not drink, each day when I eat what actually nourishes me, I take another small step away from the part of me that only wants to be numb. There are many nights that I still yearn for that smooth cool glass of wine in my hand. The warm feeling in my mouth and throat as it goes down, the glow that starts in my stomach and spreads through my body, the oblivion.

These days I keep flowers in the house, a bouquet in my bedroom. I am still overweight, but I feel good. I wear bright colors, long skirts, soft blouses. I write in my journal; I am drawing and sketching. I am teaching a class in journal writing. I moved the kitchen table into the family room next to the big window that looks out into the garden. We have a table and chairs on the deck.

The process of recovering from food and alcohol abuse has been a transition, a bridge that has taken me across to another side where my eyes are open, my senses alert.

I have learned that I can nourish myself, that it is

possible to be in control of my body, that I can meet my own needs. And nourishing myself is the only way I will be able to nourish others.

I can no longer lie back in bed with a glass of red wine and bread and butter between me and the rest of the world. I have taken a new route. I have a sense that it will have areas of great difficulty and unexpected joy. This place that I have come to is a new beginning.

—*Florinda Colavin*

Epilogue

Everything I've written about breaking free from compulsive eating is founded on my belief in the self as worthy of trust, respect and love. There are people who do not agree. They say you have to be constantly on guard against your basic tendency to act in ways that are wrong or bad. Or they may say that delusions hide you from your true inner nature and that, in your ignorance, you act according to these delusions rather than from any inner clarity.

The philosophy of breaking free stems from my experience of growth—my own and that of the hundreds of people with whom I've worked. When I am motivated by fear, the effects of what I do are temporary. But when I act out of self-trust, the roots of my behavior and attitudes are affected, and any change that results from such movement becomes well integrated into my daily life. I find it humiliating and paralyzing to be told that, if I followed my own inclinations, I would extinguish my innate wisdom and clarity—whereas I find it inspiring to affirm those qualities and allow myself the respect to become more and more of that wise and clear self.

Invariably, the people I work with have previously tried one or more disciplined approaches to weight loss, with little success. When they learn that they have a voice within them that can guide their well-being, and then when they begin listening to that voice, they become stronger, more sure of their intuitive ability to choose what satisfies them rather than what leaves them hungry.

The thrill is indescribable when, having decided long ago that your compulsive eating is hopeless, you discover that you do have the ability to choose what to eat and when, that you really don't ever have to go on another diet (it's not a lie), and that, in addition to all this, you are losing weight. It is as if you have been crawling over parched and barren land for years, have given up hope of ever finding meadows, and then suddenly you come upon green lushness and thousands of china-blue irises, pulsing and swaying to a windsong.

The physical and emotional transformations such discoveries precipitate fill me with awe. Though I recognize the cliché, I see cocoons crawl into my workshops and butterflies emerge from them. . . .

There is nothing inherently "wrong" or "right" with the breaking-free method versus the traditional, more disciplined approaches. All are aimed at encouraging the fullest potential of a human being to unfold. Some people need a more authoritarian approach than others; it works for them to be told what to do and when.

Ultimately, the decision is your own; you must do what helps you grow. And you must trust that you are wise enough to know what that is.